Monographs on Endocrinology

Volume 21

Edited by

F. Gross, Heidelberg · M. M. Grumbach, San Francisco
A. Labhart, Zürich · M. B. Lipsett, Bethesda
T. Mann, Cambridge · L. T. Samuels (†), Salt Lake City
J. Zander, München

A. E. Schindler

Hormones in Human Amniotic Fluid

With 23 Figures and 133 Tables

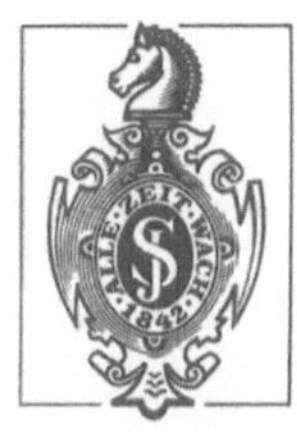

Springer-Verlag
Berlin Heidelberg New York 1982

Adolf E. Schindler, Prof. Dr. med.

Universitäts-Frauenklinik Tübingen
D-7400 Tübingen
Federal Republic of Germany

Library of Congress Cataloging in Publication Data.

Schindler, A.E (Adolf E.), 1936–. Hormones in human amniotic fluid.
(Monographs on endocrinology; v. 21)
Bibliography: p. Includes index. 1. Steroid hormones – Analysis. 2. Peptide hormones – Analysis.
3. Amniotic fluid – Analysis and chemistry. 4. Prenatal diagnosis. I. Title. II. Series.
[DNLM: 1. Amniotic fluid – Analysis. 2. Fetus – Metabolism. 3. Hormones – Analysis. W1 MO57 v. 21/WQ 210.5 S336h]
QP572.S7S34 612'.64 81-14412

ISBN-13: 978-3-642-81658-1 **e-ISBN-13: 978-3-642-81656-7**
DOI: 10.1007/ 978-3-642-81656-7

Softcover reprint of the hardcover 1st edition 1982

2127/3020-543210

Dedicated
to
My Mother

Preface

This monograph represents the first comprehensive review of hormones in human amniotic fluid and includes data published up to and including 1980. Recently, more extensive use of amniocentesis for prenatal diagnosis and evaluation of fetal lung maturation has shown that amniotic fluid hormone measurements can aid in the diagnosis of fetal and placental abnormalities.

The material is presented in two main sections dealing with steroid and protein hormones. The methods of identification and quantitation are delineated, and the findings are discussed in relation to the clinical conditions. In addition, particular attention has been directed towards up-to-date review of the sources, metabolism and transfer of human amniotic fluid hormones.

The review is intended to serve the needs of clinicians, basic scientists and students, providing detailed information on human amniotic fluid hormones in order to improve patient care and indicate possibilities for further investigations.

Tübingen, January 1982 A.E. Schindler

Contents

A. Introduction

During the past 20 years interest in amniotic fluid and its constituents has been expanding. This interest is manifold reaching from studies on the origin and regulation of amniotic fluid to inorganic and organic substances, enzymes, hormones, and cell particles. From the knowledge gained, useful clinical applications have been developed, such as intrauterine monitoring of fetal well-being or early prenatal diagnosis of fetal abnormalities.

Particularly the development of specific, sensitive, and relatively simple methods for hormone measurements in body fluids and tissues have made it possible to isolate, identify and quantitate hormones in human amniotic fluid. This was paralleled by the recognition that amniotic fluid does not represent a stagnant fluid surrounding the fetus [1] and that the fetus is not a passive occupant of this surrounding, but actively participates and cooperates with the placenta (termed fetoplacental unit) [2, 3] to create a certain "hormone milieu."

Since direct intrauterine fetal hormone measurements are not yet possible, the quantitation of hormones in amniotic fluid appeared to be a more direct approach than the determination of the hormone content in maternal blood and urine since they do not directly correlate with the endocrine function of the fetus as a whole or particular fetal organs.

It is the aim of this book to sum up the present knowledge (to the end of 1980) on hormones in human amniotic fluid from a basic scientific and clinical point of view and to delineate practical consequences gained from these studies.

B. Origin of Human Amniotic Fluid

Formation of the amnion has been reported to occur between the 7th and 8th day after ovulation from the cytotrophoblastic disk immediately adjacent to the dorsal aspect of the germ disk [4, 5]. The amniotic sac enlarges rapidly and comes into contact with the internal surface of the chorion after the 2nd month of gestation [4]. As pregnancy progresses, the amnion differentiates into five distinct layers [6].

Many theories regarding the origin of amniotic fluid have been developed [7, 8]. However, none alone could give a satisfactory answer for all phases of pregnancy. Early amniotic fluid production was considered to be due to the secretory activity of the amniotic cells since these cells show histologically secretory granules [5, 8], but during later stages of gestation the amniotic membrane becomes avascular and the maximum rate of increase in amniotic fluid (30 weeks of gestation) corresponds to a time when the amniotic cells regress; in the case of polyhydramnios, a complete absence of secretory cells has been reported [5]. According to the composition of this early fluid, the amniotic fluid is isotonic when compared to maternal and fetal plasma and therefore considered an ultrafiltrate of plasma [9]. This could explain the presence of fluid in the amniotic sac of blighted ova in which the fetus is rudimentary or absent [5], but could also be compatible with secretory activity of the amniotic epithelium. The content of lipids and proteins is low, and the fluid is compatible with the interstitial fluid of the body [9]. Therefore, in early pregnancy, amniotic fluid can be considered an extracellular space of the fetus [10].

During the course of pregnancy, amniotic fluid becomes hypotonic caused most likely by increasing amounts of fetal urine [11]. Fetal voiding was already assumed by Hippocrates, and recent studies have strongly supported this theory [12]. Fifty years ago, association between oligohydramnios and malformation of the fetal urinary tract was described, and many reports have followed [12, 13]. However, normal or excess fluid volumes have also been described in such cases [12]; one has to consider that these fetuses are abnormal also in other aspects and that this could account for the amniotic fluid volume found. In any case, the conclusion that fetal urine contributes mainly to amniotic fluid is based on a number of biochemical measurements. In early pregnancy the amount of creatinine, urea, and uric acid is similar to that found in the maternal and fetal serum [14]. These substances increase in amniotic fluid throughout pregnancy so that at term the concentration of creatinine, urea, and uric acid is about twice that of maternal and fetal serum [14a]. Measurements of creatinine and urea in fetal urine as the fetus gains in weight from 950 to 2500 g showed an increase for creatinine from 4.8 to 10.3 mg% and for urea from 69 to 172 mg% [15]. Furthermore, sodium and chloride content in amniotic fluid during early pregnancy correspond to a dialysate of maternal serum. As pregnancy proceeds, the amniotic fluid becomes hypotonic with a decrease of sodium and chloride as well as total solids [9, 14]. This corresponds to the low osmolarity of human fetal urine. Human fetal kidney function has been demonstrated at approximately the 10th to 12th week of gestation [12, 16]. Hourly fetal urine production was measured at 30 weeks to be 9.6 ml, increasing until term to 27.3 ml [17, 18]. At term, the human fetus seems to be able to void more than 450 ml/24 h.

Proper function of the fetal kidneys has been indicated by studies on fetal urine glucose [19] and excretion of different antibiotics [20] as well as by other studies [21–23]. The fetal urine is not a dialysate of fetal plasma. The fetal kidneys have the capability to excrete certain substances preferentially and to retain others. This is of importance in regard to steroids in amniotic fluid.

Another major factor influencing amniotic fluid volume is fetal swallowing. Active deglutition of amniotic fluid has been believed for a long time and subsequently demonstrated in different ways [5, 12, 18]. At term, the human fetus seems to be able to swallow up to 500 ml a day [24]; in the case of hydramnios, deglutition appears to be reduced [25], a finding that would explain hydramnios in fetuses with esophageal atresia [12, 26].

The significance of amniotic fluid regulation by the human fetal respiratory tract has not yet been clarified [5, 12]. Studies with labeled erythrocytes at least indicate increasing amounts of aspirated amniotic fluid as pregnancy progresses [27] and near term reach about 200 ml/kg/day [28].

The pathway of water and/or solids across the fetal skin probably changes throughout pregnancy as the skin changes its structure [5, 12]. Again, definite quantitative data are not available.

The total turnover of water and solutes to and from amniotic fluid is subject to different pathways and many factors involving the maternal and fetal compartment, placenta, and amniotic membranes. The exchange can occur in the following ways:

1) Between amniotic fluid and maternal circulation
   a) Directly via amnion and chorion
   b) Indirectly via placenta
   c) Indirectly via umbilical cord
   d) Indirectly via fetus
2) Between amniotic fluid and fetus
   a) Volume addition by fetal urine
   b) Volume reduction by fetal deglutition, aspiration and probably by fetal skin absorption.

In general, osmotic and hydrostatic forces act upon the exchange processes, leading to a certain amount of water circulating from the mother to the fetus, amniotic fluid, and back to the mother [29]. It should be kept in mind that these factors can in turn be modified, for instance, by maternal diseases [30]. It was demonstrated that the water of amniotic fluid is completely replaced every 2.9 h.

Studies with labeled compounds indicated a transfer of water between amniotic fluid and mother at a constant rate of 468 ml/h [12]. This, however, is molecular diffusion and must be differentiated from bulk flow, which recently was calculated for water across the human fetal membranes to be 34–83 ml/day [31]. The effectiveness of water transport of the membranes in turn can be modified by constituents within the fluid, such as prolactin, which increases throughout pregnancy [32] and appears to specifically regulate the water transport across the human amnion at term [33]. Normally, all these processes terminate in a dynamic steady state, leading to an increase of the average volume of amniotic fluid of 30 ml at 10 weeks gestation, with a maximum of 1,000 ml at 38 weeks, 800 ml at term, and a decrease thereafter—in some cases, even to a complete lack of amniotic fluid [5, 9, 12, 34].

Studies with five different proteins (serum albumin, serum γG, serum γA, HCG, and HGH), led to the conclusion that they are cleared from the amniotic fluid at similar rates despite marked differences in the molecular weights and metabolic functions of these proteins. It was calculated that on the average two-thirds or more of the amniotic fluid volume is cleared daily of protein in the presence of a living fetus, over 80 % of this apparently by fetal swallowing; the daily clearance of amniotic fluid averaged 342 ml in the absence of labor and 554 ml during labor. Fetal urine was the apparent source of a large fraction of γG found in amniotic fluid, but fetal serum contributed less than 5 % of the albumin and little or none of the γA present in amniotic fluid. The volume of amniotic fluid swallowed by the fetus tended to vary directly with the volume of fluid in the amniotic cavity, which could serve to stabilize amniotic fluid volume [35]. Recently, current concepts of amniotic fluid dynamics have been reviewed [35a].

C. Origin and Regulation of Steroids in Human Amniotic Fluid

Theoretically, an influx of steroids into amniotic fluid could occur via the umbilical cord or the placenta, according to concentration gradients. Up to the present time, such pathways have not yet been proved. Therefore, the main access of steroids into the amniotic fluid is by fetal urine. This conclusion is based upon identical steroid patterns in both biologic fluids [34].

Elimination of steroids from amniotic fluid is possible in different ways:

1) Uptake through fetal skin [36]
2) Deglutition of amniotic fluid and absorption through the bowel [37]
3) Aspiration of amniotic fluid; according to the available experimental evidence, this pathway appears to be of no major importance [36, 37]
4) Transport through the amniotic membranes and elimination into the maternal circulation [38, 39]

The latter mechanism is dependent upon the type of conjugation of the steroid molecule. The passage of nonconjugated estrogens occurs freely. Estrogen sulfates are hydrolyzed and then the transfer accomplished, while estrogen glucoronides transverse slowly without being hydrolyzed [38].

Two types of pathways for elimination of steroids from amniotic fluid can be postulated:

1) Between amniotic fluid and maternal compartment
2) Between amniotic fluid and fetus

The quantitative importance of these pathways has not yet been established.

The steroid content of amniotic fluid might also be modified through synthesis and metabolism of steroids in the amniotic membranes as shown by a number of investigators [40–47]; of the protein hormones, prolactin could be derived from the amniotic membranes [46, 48–52, 52a].

D. Methods of Isolation and Identification of Steroids in Human Amniotic Fluid

I. C_{30}, C_{29}, and C_{28} Steroids

In 1968 isolation and identification of these steroids were carried out by combined thin-layer chromatography (TLC), gas-liquid chromatography (GLC), and gas-liquid chromatography-mass spectrometry (GLC-MS), indicating that about 2% of the total sterol content in amniotic fluid consisted of C_{30}, C_{29}, and C_{28} steroids [53]. The lanosterols (lanosterol, Δ^8-lanosterol, Δ^4-lanosterol, Δ^5-lanosterol) were major components compared to methostenols, of which the Δ^8-isomer dominated. The precursor of lanosterol, squalene, was recently identified by GLC-MS in amniotic fluid [54] and described as representing 72%–78% of the hydrocarbons of the lipids in amniotic fluid [55].

II. C_{27} Steroids

1. **Cholesterol** (cholest-5-ene-3β-ol)

Isolation and identification of amniotic fluid cholesterol was first reported in 1963 after petroleum ether extraction, digitonin fractionation twice before and after alkaline wash, crystallization of the free and acetylated form combined with melting point determinations, and infrared spectrum analysis. A concentration of 40 mg/liter was estimated. The free form and an esterified form were described [56]. Cholesterol was also identified by combined TLC, GLC, and GLC-MS as trimethylsilyl (TMSI) derivative [53] and recently confirmed [54].

2. **Cholestanol** (5α-cholestane-3β-ol)

This steroid was isolated by combined TLC, GLC, and GLC-MS [56].

3. **Δ^7-Cholestenol** (5α-cholest-7-ene-3β-ol) **and Δ^8-Cholestenol** (5α-cholest-8-ene-3β-ol)

Identification of these compounds was done [56] by TLC, GLC, and GLC-MS.

4. **7-Dehydrocholesterol** (cholest-5,7-dione-3β-ol) **and Desmosterol** (cholest-5,24-dione-3,5-ol)

These substances were identified in amniotic fluid by TLC, GLC, and GLC-MS [56].

III. Δ^5-C_{21} Steroids

1. **Pregnenolone** (pregn-5-ene-20-one-3β-ol)

An attempt was made to isolate and identify pregnenolone from 4,000 ml normal amniotic fluid at term, but this steroid could not be detected [57].

2. **16α-Hydroxypregnenolone** (preg-5-ene-20-one-3β,16α-diol)

Identification was done from a pool of 4 liters normal amniotic fluid at term by celite column chromatography, TLC, GLC, and GLC-MS as diacetate and TMSI derivative using internal standard techniques. The concentration was found to be 119.0 μg/liter [57].

3. **17α-Hydroxypregnenolone** (preg-5-ene-20-one-3β,17α-diol)

This steroid was first measured by a specific radioimmunoassay after celite column chromatography [58]. Other studies of isolation and identification of this steroid in human amniotic fluid have not been published.

4. **Pregn-5-ene-3β,20α-diol**

This steroid was identified in the disulfate fraction after Sephadex LH-20 column chromatography, GLC, and GLC-MS as TMSI derivative in a concentration of 22 μg/liter expressed as free steroid [59].

5. **Pregn-5-ene-3β,17α,20α-triol**

This steroid was isolated from normal amniotic fluid as the disulfate by Sephadex LH-20 column chromatography, GLC, and GLC-MS as TMSI derivative with a concentration of 26 μg/liter expressed as free steroid [59].

6. **21-Hydroxypregnenolone** (pregn-5-ene-20-one-3β,21-diol)

This steroid was isolated from amniotic fluid obtained from normal pregnancies at term within the disulfate fraction by Sephadex LH-20 column chromatography, silicic acid column chromatography, TLC, GLC, and GLC-MS as TMSI derivative and O-methyloxime trimethylsilyl ether derivative on 3% QF-1 and 2.2% SE-30 column. A concentration of 122 μg/liter expressed as free steroid was found [60].

7. **Pregn-5-ene-3β,20α,21-triol**

Isolation from the disulfate fraction after Sephadex LH-20 and silicic acid column chromatography, TLC, GLC (column coated with 3% QF-1 or 2.2% SE-30), and GLC-MS as TMSI derivative and O-isopropylidene trimethylsilyl ether derivative was accomplished, and a concentration of 12 μg/liter expressed as free steroid was found [60].

IV. Δ^4-C_{21} Steroids

1. **Progesterone** (pregn-4-ene-3,20-dione)

A first attempt to isolate and quantitate progesterone from human amniotic fluid was reported in 1956. After extraction and paper chromatography, the steroid was verified by infrared spectrometry [61]. Later, progesterone (Prog) was identified from 41 samples of normal human amniotic fluid using celite column chromatography, TLC and GLC, with columns coated with 1% SE-30, 1% SE/1% QF-1, or 1% OV-1. Final identification was done by GLC-MS on a 1% SE-30 column. The concentration of Prog in 4 liters normal amniotic fluid was 39.4 μg/liter without correction for procedural losses [57]. From another pool of 740 ml normal amniotic fluid at term, progesterone was also isolated by celite column chromatography, TLC, GLC, and GLC-MS using internal standard techniques. A concentration of 52 μg/liter was found [62].

2. **16α-Hydroxyprogesterone** (pregn-4-ene-3,20-dione-16α-ol)

This steroid was identified in a pool of 740 ml normal amniotic fluid at term after enzyme hydrolysis with β-glucoronidase/aryl sulfatase, celite column chromatography, TLC, GLC as TMSI derivative, and GLC-MS. A concentration of 130 μ/liter was measured using internal standard techniques [62].

3. **17α-Hydroxyprogesterone** (pregn-4-ene-3,20-dione-17α-ol)

This steroid was first measured by specific radioimmunoassay after addition of paper chromatography prior to quantitation. Identical results were obtained with this procedure by triplicates with and without additional paper chromatography [0.21 ± 0.01 (SEM) μg/liter and 1.98 ± 0.02 (SEM) μg/liter, respectively] [63].

4. **Cortisol** (compound F, pregn-4-ene-3,20-dione-11β,17α,21-triol)

The first report on cortisol in amniotic fluid was published in 1954 [64]. The compound was isolated by paper chromatography, however, only in samples from diabetic pregnancies [64].

In normal amniotic fluid, the isolation procedure for cortisol was reasonably good using two paper chromatograms, acetylation, and NaOH-fluorescence reaction [65]. In a similar manner, cortisol was also identified in human amniotic fluid from normal and complicated pregnancies describing the presence of the free and conjugated moiety [56]. Studies of the free, sulfate, and glucoronide fraction resulted in the isolation of cortisol from the free and sulfate fraction after respective enzyme hydrolysis, paper chromatography (PC), TLC, acetylation, and crystallization using double isotope-derivative techniques [66, 67].

5. **6β-Hydroxycortisol** (pregn-4-ene-3,20-dione-6β,11β,17α,21-tetrol)

This steroid was identified in amniotic fluid using the following procedures:

ultraviolet absorption in alcohol, reaction with blue tetrazolium, fluorescence with NaOH, mobility in two paper chromatography systems, absorption spectrum in concentrated sulfuric acid, chromatographic mobility after acetylation, and mobility after reduction using sodium bismuthate [68].

6. 6β,20β-Dihydroxycortisol (pregn-4-ene-3-one-6β,11β,17α,20β,21-pentol)

The identification was based upon the following criteria: ultraviolet absorption in ethanol, reaction with blue tetrazolium, chromatographic mobility after sodium bismuthate oxidation in two chromatographic systems, and identical Rf values after acetylation, further oxidation, and reduction after acetylation [69].

7. 11-Deoxycortisol (compound S, pregn-4-ene-3,20-dione-17α,21-diol)

This steroid has only been measured by radioimmunoassay using dichloromethane extraction and Sephadex LH-20 column chromatography [70, 70a]. Further isolation and identification studies are not available.

8. 21-Deoxycortisol (pregn-4-ene-3,20-dione-11β,17α-diol)

Only one report on this steroid in human amniotic fluid was found [70a]. The measurements were done by RIA. Isolation and identification studies have not been reported.

9. Cortisone (compound E, pregn-4-ene-3,11,20-trione-17α,21-diol)

This steroid was identified in ways similar to those described for cortisol [56, 64–67]. It was found in the unconjugated form, but also as glucoronide [56], while others have found conjugation only as the sulfate [66, 67].

10. 6β,20β-Dihydroxycortisone (pregn-4-ene-3,11-dione-6β,17α,20β,21-tetrol)

The identification procedure was as follows: ultraviolet absorption in ethanol, reaction with blue tetrazolium, paper chromatographic mobility before and after oxidation with sodium bismuthate and after acetylation, and oxidation as well as reduction [69].

11. Corticosterone (compound B, pregn-4-ene-3,20-dione-11β,21-diol)

The first isolation of this steroid in human amniotic fluid was described in 1971. Paper chromatography, acetylation, double isotope-derivative techniques, and crystallization were utilized to verify this steroid in the free and sulfate fraction [66, 67].

12. 11-Dehydrocorticosterone (compound A, pregn-4-ene-3,11,20-trione-21-ol)

The procedure of identification and quantitation was similar to that described for corticosterone. The steroid was also found in the free and sulfate fraction [66, 67].

13. 11-Deoxycorticosterone (DOC, pregn-4-ene-3,20-dione-21-ol)

This steroid was identified only in the sulfate fraction [66].

14. Aldosterone (pregn-4-ene-3,20-dime-11β,21-diol-18-al)

Aldosterone was determined in amniotic fluid by radioimmunoassay [71, 71a]. A concentration of 1–10 μg/liter was found. Further isolation and identification procedures have not been published.

V. Pregnane Steroids

1. Pregnanolone (5β-pregnane-20-one-3α-ol)

The steroid was found in the glucoronide fraction from amniotic fluid at term after Sephadex LH-20 column chromatography, hydrolysis with β-glucuronidase, silicic acid column chromatography, and GLC-MS as TMSI and MO-TMSI derivative. The amount was calculated to be 43 μg/liter [72].

Recently, this steroid was also identified and measured in the glucuronide fraction in term amniotic fluid after amberlite XAD-7 chromatography, two-step hydrolysis, silica gel column chromatography, and glass capillary gas chromatography [73]. In a pool of amniotic fluid, the concentration was 60 μg/liter and in 20 samples the concentration was 43 μg/liter [73].

2. Pregnanediol (5β-pregnane-3α,20α-diol)

In 1954 an attempt was made to identify pregnanediol in amniotic fluid [74]. Isolation, identification, and quantitation of pregnanediol were first accomplished in 1959 [75]. A sample of 4.8 liters of amniotic fluid was taken from a pregnancy with an anencephalic fetus and twice the amniotic fluid was obtained from normal pregnancies. Pregnanediol was not found in the unhydrolyzed fraction. After acid hydrolysis following extraction, alkaline partition, alumina column chromatography, acetylation and crystallization from benzene were carried out. The compound was identified by ultraviolet spectrum analysis of the free and acetylated form. A melting point analysis was not done because of impurities. The concentration was estimated to be about 400 μg/liter.

A more subtle isolation procedure was published in 1968 [57]. Enzyme hydrolysis with 1,000 IU glucuronidase and 500 IU sulfatase/ml was done with 4 liters of normal amniotic fluid and after addition of tritium-labeled 5β-pregnane-3α,20α-diol extracted with ethyl acetate followed by celite column chromatography and TLC in two different systems separating Δ^5-pregnene-3β,20α-diol and 5α-pregnane-3β,20α-diol, then GLC as trimethylsilyl ether and diacetate derivatives on columns coated with 1% SE-30, 1% SE-30/1% QF-1, or 1% OV-1. Final identification was obtained for both derivatives by GLC-MS on a column coated with 1% SE-30. The amount isolated was 412.0 μg/liter with a 70.8% recovery leading to a concentration of total pregnane-diol in normal amniotic fluid of 145.4 μg/liter. In amniotic fluid from early and midgestation, pregnanediol could be identified in the disulfate fraction after extraction with acetone/ethanol, Sephadex LH-20 column chromatography, solvolysis, silicic acid chromatography, GLC, and GLC-MS as TMSI derivatives. Without correction for losses, 11.9 μg/liter were reported [76].

As glucuronide using Sephadex LH-20 column chromatography, hydrolysis with β-glucuronidase, silicic acid column chromatography, and GLC-MS as TMSI derivative, a concentration of 281 μg/liter was found [72]. Using amberlite XAD-7 chromatography, fractional hydrolysis, silica gel column chromatography, and capillary glass column gas chromatography, the concentration in a pool of amniotic fluid was found to be 263 μg/liter [73].

3. 5α-Pregnane-3α,20α-diol and 5α-Pregnane-3β,20α-diol

Both steroids were identified from the sulfate fraction in amniotic fluid from early to mid- and late pregnancy [59, 60, 76], including Sephadex LH-20 column chromatography, solvolysis, silicic acid column chromatography, GLC and GLC-MS as TMSI derivatives. The concentration rose from 7.1 and 4.1 μg/liter, respectively, in early and midpregnancy to 36 and 38/49 μg/liter respectively, in late pregnancy [59, 60, 76].

4. 5α-Pregnane-20-one-3α,21-diol

This steroid was isolated from the disulfate fraction in a manner similar to that described above, and a concentration of 18 μg/liter was found [60].

5. 5α-Pregnane-20-one-3α,16α-diol and 5β-Pregnane-20-one-3β,16α-diol

Both steroids were isolated from the glucuronide fraction of normal amniotic fluid after Sephadex LH-20 column chromatography, hydrolysis with β-glucuronidase, silicic acid column chromatography, GLC, and GLC-MS as MO-TMSI derivatives. The total quantity of both was 223 μg/liter [72].

Recently, 5α-pregnane-20-one 3α,16α-diol glucuronide was isolated and quantitated in amniotic fluid at term by amberlite XAD-7 chromatography, two-step hydrolysis, silica gel chromatography, and glass capillary gas chromatography. In a pool of amniotic fluid, a concentration of 154 μg/liter was found [73].

6. 5β-Pregnane-20-one-3α,6α-diol

This steroid was isolated as glucuronide after Sephadex LH-20 column chromatography, hydrolysis, β-glucuronidase, silicic acid column chromatography, GLC as TMSI and MO-TMSI derivatives, and GLC-MS; a quantity of 166 μg/liter was found [72]. A further isomer was also detected, but not completely identified [72]. The presence of this steroid as glucuronide in amniotic fluid was recently reported, and a concentration of 52 μg/liter found [73].

7. **Pregnanetriol** (5β-pregnane-3α,17α,20α-triol)

The first isolation and identification were described in 1965, including enzyme hydrolysis, alumina column chromatography, thin-layer chromatography, sodium periodate oxidation, and treatment with Zimmermann reagent combined with TLC [77]. More recently, this steroid was isolated from the glucoronide fraction by Sephadex LH-20 column chromatography, hydrolysis, with β-glucuronidase, silicic acid column chromatography, and GLC-MS as TMSI derivative. A concentration of 145 μg/liter has been found [72].

In a follow-up study, the glucuronide moiety of this steroid was measured in a pool of amniotic fluid at term to be 45 μg/liter [73]. In contrast, using a radioactively labeled internal standard technique, differential extraction, and hydrolysis, it could be demonstrated that pregnanetriol is normally found in the sulfate fraction, and in abnormal conditions this steroid is also present in the free fraction [78].

8. **5α-Pregnane-3α,20α,21-triol**

This steroid was identified by GLC-MS as TMSI and O-isopropylidene trimethylsilyl ether derivative from the disulfate fraction. Only trace amounts were detected [60].

9. **5α-Pregnane-3β,16α,20α-triol**

The steroid has been found in the glucuronide fraction of amniotic fluid after Sephadex LH-20 column chromatography, hydrolysis with β-glucuronidase, and GLC-MS as TMSI derivative. A quantity of 87 μg/liter was found [72].

10. **Tetrahydrocortisol** (THF, 5β-pregnane-20-one-3α,11β,17α,21-terol), **Tetrahydrocortisone** (THE, 5β-pregnane-11,20-dione-3α,17α,21-triol), **and Tetrahydro-11-dehydrocorticosterone** (THA, 5β-pregnane-11,20-dione-3α,21-diol)

Isolation and identification were done by repeated chromatography as the free compound and as acetate as well as after oxidation and crystallization to a constant isotope ratio. These steroids were isolated from the glucuronide fraction [66, 67]. After enzyme hydrolysis with β-glucuronidase and arylsulfatase, column chromatography (DEAE-Sephadex A-25, Amberlite-XAD-2, Silica gel), and high-pressure liquid chromatography, THF and THE were identified and measured by capillary gas chromatography as O-methoxine trimethylsilyl ethers. A concentration of 290 ± 28 (SEM) μg/nmol creatinine for THF and 1,022 ± 266 (SEM) μg/nmol creatinine for THE were found in human amniotic fluid near term [433].

11. **Tetrahydro-11-deoxycortisol** (THS, 5β-pregnane-20-one-3α,17α,21-triol)

Only data obtained by a specific radioimmunoassay are available from this steroid in human amniotic fluid [79]. Specific isolation and identification procedures have not been reported [79].

12. **6α-OH-Tetrahydroxycortisol** (6-OH-THF, 5β-pregnane-20-one-3α,6α,17α,21-pentol), **6α-OH-Tetrahydroxycortisone** (6-OH-THE, 5β-pregnane-11,20-dione-3α,6α,17α,21-tetrol), **6α-OH-Allotetrahydroxycortisol** (6-OH-ATHF, 5α-pregnane-20-one-3α,6α,11β,17α,21-pentol), **6α-OH-Allotetrahydroxycortisone** (6-OH-ATHE, 5α-pregnane-11,20-dione-3α,6α,17α,21-tetrol), **6α-OH-20α-Cortolone** (5β-pregnane-11-one-3α,6α,17α,20α,21-pentol), **and 6α-OH-20β-Cortolone** (5β-pregnane-11-one-3α,6α,17α,20β,21-pentol)

All the steroids were identified and measured after enzyme hydrolysis with β-glucuronidase and arylsulfatase, column chromatography (DEAE-Sephadex A-25, Amberlite XAD-2, Silica gel), high-pressure liquid chromatography, and GLC-MS [433]. In a few samples near term, the following concentrations were found (mean ± SEM μg/nmol cratinine): 6-OH-THF 175 ± 25, 6-OH-THE 211 ±18, 6-OH-ATHF 17.3 ± 4.8, 6-OH-ATHE 20 (one case), 6α-OH-20α-cortolone 42.3 ± 7.9, 6α-OH-20β-cortolone 111 ± 46 [433].

VI. Δ^5-C_{19} Steroids

1. **Dehydroepiandrosterone** (D, androst-5-ene-17-one-3β-ol)

In 1964, D was mentioned to be present in human amniotic fluid [80]. Identification of the steroid was done 4 years later by enzyme hydrolysis, celite column chromatography, TLC, GLC, and GLC-MS as TMSI derivative, calculating a concentration of 8.3 μg/liter [57].

2. Androst-5-ene-3β,17α-diol

This steroid was first identified in amniotic fluid in the disulfate fraction after Sephadex LH-20 column chromatography, solvolysis, silicic acid column chromatography, GLC as TMSI derivative, and GLC-MS. Concentrations of 224 and 236 μg/liter were found [59, 60]. It was also identified in the disulfate fraction of amniotic fluid of early and midpregnancy in a similar manner where a concentration of 6.3 μg/liter was found [76].

3. Androst-5-ene-3β,17β-diol

This steroid was identified also as disulfate using the above-mentioned procedure [59, 60]. The concentration at term reached 42 and 56 μg/liter [59, 60] and in early and midpregnancy 2.6 μg/liter [76].

4. **16α-Hydroxydehydroepiandrosterone** (androst-5-ene-17-one-3β,16α-diol)

This steroid was first identified in 1968 after enzyme hydrolysis, celite column chromatography, TLC, GLC as TMSI derivative and diacetate, and GLC-MS with a concentration of 797.7 μg/liter [57]. The steroid was also isolated by others in a similar manner [81]. In the disulfate fraction, this steroid was isolated and a quantity of 48 μg/liter found at term [59]. A small amount was also detected in the monosulfate fraction [59]. A concentration of 8.2 μg/liter was found in early and midpregnancy [76].

5. 16β-Hydroxydehydroepiandrosterone (androst-5-ene-17-one-3β,16β-diol)

This compound has been identified in the disulfate fraction at term as well as in early and midpregnancy in a concentration of 88 and 2.3 μg/liter, respectively [59, 76] and reported in pooled amniotic fluid as sulfate in a concentration of 30 μg/liter [82].

6. 16,18-Dihydroxydehydroepiandrosterone

This compound has been isolated and quantitated by GLC and GLC-MS [82]. The concentration as sulfate in a pool of amniotic fluid was 40 μg/liter [82].

7. 16-Ketoandrostenediol (16-keto-A, Androst-5-ene-16-one-3β,17β-diol)

The first isolation was accomplished from 4 liters of normal amniotic fluid in 1968 [57] after enzyme hydrolysis, celite column chromatography, TLC, GLC as diacetate and TMSI derivative, and GLC-MS. A concentration of 575 μg/liter was isolated and with a similar procedure 1,100 μg/liter [81]. Small amounts were detected in the disulfate fraction at term and in early and midpregnancy with 6 and 15 μg/liter, respectively [59, 81].

8. Androstenetriol (A-triol, androst-5-ene-3β,16α,17β-triol)

The presence of this steroid was first described in normal amniotic fluid at term after enzyme hydrolysis, celite column chromatography, TLC, GLC as TMSI and acetate derivative, and GLC-MS [57], revealing a concentration of 48 μg/liter [57].

9. Androst-5-ene-3β,16β,17α-triol

This isomer was identified in the disulfate fraction by means of Sephadex LH-20 column chromatography, solvolysis, silicic acid column chromatography, GLC as TMSI derivative, and GLC-MS; a concentration of 38 μg/liter measured [60]. As glucuronide, this steroid was isolated and identified using Sephadex LH-20 column chromatography, enzyme hydrolysis with β-glucuronidase, silica gel column chromatography, GLC, and GLC-MS as TMSI derivative. Only trace amounts were detected in human amniotic fluid at term [72].

VII. Δ^4-C_{19} Steroids

1. Δ^4-Androstenedione (androst-4-ene-3,17-dione)

The presence of this steroid was indicated in a study published in 1964 [80], but only recently has this steroid been measured by specific radioimmunoassay (RIA), in amniotic fluid [83–87]. Isolation and identification by GLC-MS or other specific means have not been reported.

2. **Testosterone** (androst-4-ene-3-one-17β-ol)

Testosterone was first described in amniotic fluid pools [88, 89]. Later, testosterone was isolated by column-, paper-, and thin-layer chromatography and measurement with a competitive protein binding method [90]. Isolation and identification by GLC-MS or other specific means have not been reported. A number of studies using radioimmunoassays have been published to date [83–85, 87, 91–102].

VIII. Androstane Steroids

1. **Dihydrotestosterone** (DHT, 5α-androstan-3-one-17β-ol)

One study reported that DHT is not detectable in amniotic fluid [98]. More recently, DHT was measured by RIA in amniotic fluid but could only be detected in pregnancies with male fetuses [87].

2. **5α-Androstan-17-one-3α,18-diol**

This steroid was isolated from amniotic fluid of anencephalic fetuses and tentative identification was made by GLC as TMSI derivative and GLC-MS [103].

IX. C_{18} Steroids

1. **Estrone** (E_1, estra-1,3,5(10)-triene-17-one-3-ol)

Estrone was first measured by methods used for tissue, blood, or urine estrogen determinations [104–108]. Identification was done by GLC and GLC-MS [81].

2. **16α-Hydroxyestrone** (estra-1,3,5(10)-triene-17-one-3,16α-diol)

Besides GLC evidence, identification was substantiated by column and paper chromatography as well as GLC-MS as TMSI derivative [81]. The concentration ranged from 18–46 μg/liter in three pools [81]; 2.7 μg/liter were measured as free moiety and 24.7 μg/liter as conjugates in seven pooled samples [109].

3. **16β-Hydroxyestrone** (estra-1,3,5(10)-triene-17-one-3,16β-diol)

In addition to identical retention time on GLC, the isolated compound was also subjected to Girard separation, solvent partition, chromatography on partially deactivated alumina, and two paper chromatographic systems. The mass spectrum of the di-TMSI derivative, however, was contaminated and therefore no definite conclusions could be drawn [81]. One measurement was carried out, and the values are possibly overestimated because of contamination resulting in 31 μg/liter [81]. In conjugated form, 17.8 μg/liter were found later [109].

4. **15α-Hydroxyestrone** (estra-1,3,5(10)-triene-17-one-3,15α-diol)

Tentative identification was made for this steroid in amniotic fluid. The isolated substance behaved identically with the reference standard on GLC, after Girard separation, solvent partition, and paper chromatography in two systems. The mass spectrum of the di-TMSI derivative was somewhat contaminated with another steroid and therefore conclusive identification not achieved [81]. A single determination revealed a concentration of 7 μg/liter. Separate estimations of the free and conjugated form revealed 1.0 and 5.5 μg/liter, respectively [109].

5. **2-Methoxyestrone** (estra-1,3,5(10)-triene-17-one-2,3-driol-2-methylether)

The accumulated evidence does indicate that this steroid is present in amniotic fluid; however, this does not allow definite identification [81, 109]. A concentration between 0.2 and 0.3 μg/liter in three pools was measured [81].

6. **Estradiol-17β** (E_2, estra-1,3,5(10)-triene-3,17β-diol)

Similar to estrone, this steroid was first measured in amniotic fluid by various methods [104–108]; later identification was established by GLC and GLC-MS [81].

7. **16-Ketoestradiol** (estra-1,3,5(10)-triene-16-one-3,17β-diol)

This steroid was definitely identified by GLC-MS after a thorough work-up [81]. The concentration in three pools ranged between 16 and 23 μg/liter [81].

8. **11-Dehydroestradiol-17α**

This compound was found after extensive isolation procedures and identified by GLC-MS; 2.0 μg/liter were found in conjugated form [109].

9. **Estriol** (E_3, estra-1,3,5(10)-triene-3,16α,17β-triol)

Estriol was first determined by methods used for tissue, blood, and urine estrogen measurements [104–108, 110]. It was later identified after enzyme hydrolysis using celite column chromatography, TLC, GLC, and GLC-MS as TMSI derivative [57]. This was confirmed in a similar way by others [81].

10. 16-Epiestriol (estra-1,3,5(10)-triene-3,16β,17β-triol)

Identification of this steroid was accomplished using Girard separation, solvent partition, acetonide derivative formation, GLC, and GLC-MS [81]. A concentration range of 5–17 μg/liter was found in three pools [81].

11. 17-Epiestriol (estra-1,3,5(10)-triene-3,16α,17β-triol)

The identification procedure was nearly identical to 16-epiestriol, and amounts between 1.6 and 4.2 μg/liter were measured in three pools [81].

12. Estetrol (E_4, estra-1,3,5(10)-triene-3,15α,16α,17β-tetrol)

Identification was first obtained using enzyme hydrolysis, celite column chromatography, TLC, and GLC as acetate and TMSI derivative. Final confirmation was obtained by GLC-MS [57]. In a similar approach, the steroid was also identified by others [81].

E. Quantitation of Steroids in Human Amniotic Fluid

I. C_{30}, C_{29}, and C_{28} Steroids

Except for the identification studies reported earlier [53], further reports on the quantitation of such steroids in human amniotic fluid were not found.

A recent study on squalene indicating a steep rise at 39–40 weeks of gestation for this compound should be pointed out. The clinical usefulness for evaluating fetal maturity together with the cholesterol level is under discussion [54].

II. C_{27} Steroids

1. Cholesterol

a) Normal Pregnancies

Only a limited number of determinations have been carried out so far using a variety of methods (Table 1). Two sets of data emerge (Table 1). Methods using specific means of purification and separation (Drafta, personal communication) [116] do report concentrations about ten times lower than those obtained by spectrophotometry alone [112, 113] or autoanalyzer techniques [114, 115, 117]. The latter results are comparable to earlier reports [118]. It is most likely that the lower values obtained by GLC, for instance, reflect the true cholesterol concentration in amniotic fluid.

Some of the results do not indicate changes of the amniotic fluid content according to the weeks of gestation [54, 112, 116, 119], while data from other studies led to the conclusion that there is an increase of cholesterol in amniotic fluid as pregnancy progresses toward term [120]. Furthermore, our own data indicate that sex differences are not present [115].

b) Complicated Pregnancies

In complicated pregnancies, it has to be taken into account whether clear amniotic fluid is present or not [113] since meconium or blood-contaminated fluid appears to contain significantly ($P < 0.01 - < 0.001$) more cholesterol [113, 117]. Looking at certain clinically abnormal conditions, Anton et al. [113] found cholesterol elevations in amniotic fluid when compared to the normal value of 41.4 µg/liter: preeclampsia (n = 15) 77.6 mg/liter, prolonged pregnancy (n = 11) 111.3 mg/liter, threatened intrauterine asphyxia (n = 13) 125.8 ng/liter, intrauterine fetal death (n = 3) 102.7 mg/liter, Rh incompatibility (n = 4) 55.3 mg/liter and placental insufficiency of unknown etiology (n = 11) 168 mg/liter.

Table 1. Cholesterol in normal human amniotic fluid

Weeks of gestation	No. of samples	Cholesterol (mg/100 ml)		Method	Ref.
		Range	Mean ± SEM		
Preterm	10	1.8–10.0	5.0 ± 0.7	Spectro-photometry	111
At term	38	7.0–19.5	14.1 ± 0.5		
31	5	0– 25	15	Spectro-photometry	112
35	5	0–100	34		
36	6	0– 20	19		
37	15	0– 75	17		
38	18	0– 25	9		
39	33	0–300	23		
40	41	0– 52	14		
41	62	0– 65	13		
42	15	0– 45	13		
43	8	0– 75	16		
Near term	26	1.3– 94	4.1 ± 0.3	Spectro-photometry	113
9–24	60	2 – 60	19.6	Autoanalyzer	114
29–37	8	4 – 14	8.1 ± 1.4	Autoanalyzer	115
38–42	80	1 – 34	11.7 ± 0.9		
12–17.9	3	1.4–1.8	1.6 ± 0.08	Gas chromato-graphy	116
18–20.9	3	1.1–1.3	1.2 ± 0.05		
27–29.9	4	1.6–3.9	2.5 ± 0.35		
30–32.9	8	0.5–1.1	0.9 ± 0.11		
33–35.9	16	0.6–3.4	1.4 ± 0.21		
36–38.9	23	0.7–2.8	1.3 ± 0.14		
39–41.9	33	0.7–4.6	1.6 ± 0.14		
42	8	1.1–3.8	2.0 ± 0.26		
36–40	15	0.2–2.7	1.3 ± 0.19	Thin-layer chromato-graphy – Spectro-photometry	(Drafta, personal communi-cation)

The range is very wide and therefore no clear cutoff point between normal and abnormal values can be defined. Anton et al. [113] do conclude that using their method a level above 70 mg/liter might be indicative of feto-placental malfunction.

2. Other C_{27} Steroids

Besides the data indicated in the previous chapter on identification of steroids, no serial measurements of such steroids have been reported.

III. Δ^5-C_{21} Steroids

1. Pregnenolone

Although pregnenolone could not be identified from a pool of 4,000 ml of normal human amniotic fluid at term [57], recent measurements with RIA techniques indicated that the unconjugated moiety of the steroid is present in amniotic fluid between the 12th and 20th week of gestation at a concentration of 1.88 μg/liter. Sex differences were not observed [84].

2. 16α-Hydroxypregnenolone (16 OH-Preg)

Near term, the total 16 OH-Preg content was determined to be 119 μg/liter [57], and the sulfate fraction of the steroid was quantitated with 70 μg/liter [82]. In the sulfate and sulfoglucuronide fraction of pooled amniotic fluid at term, the concentration was found to be 46 μg/liter and in 20 individual samples to be 52 ± 8.7 (SEM) μg/liter [73].

In three cases with placental sulfatase deficiency, a mean concentration of 250 μg/liter was reported with a range of 10–30,130 μg/liter [82]; in two cases with anencephalic fetuses, the values for the sulfate and sulfoglucuronide fraction were 15 and 16 μg/liter [73].

3. 17α-Hydroxypregnenolone (17 OH-Preg)

a) Normal Pregnancies

The level of unconjugated 17 OH-Preg in the amniotic fluid of patients not in labor at term was 0.8 ± 0.1 (SEM) ng/ml (range 0.3–1.4) and similar to the data of patients undergoing elective cesarean section [58]. The values at midgestation were significantly higher ($P < 0.05$): 1.5 ± 0.3 ng/ml. The sulfate fraction at midgestation was 2.0 ± 0.2 ng/ml and at term in patients not in labor 3.6 ± 0.7 ng/ml, which was not significantly different from that of 6.4 ± 0.7 ng/ml observed in patients undergoing elective cesarean section [58].

b) Complicated Pregnancies

In congenital adrenal hyperplasia of the fetus due to 21-hydroxylase deficiency, the concentration of 17 OH-Preg was not found to be different from normal [121]. This steroid could perhaps be valuable in diagnosing congenital adrenal hyperplasia due to 3β-hydroxysteroid dehydrogenase deficiency [121]. In anencephaly, however, this steroid was undetectable (< 0.1 ng/ml), which was also the case for the sulfoconjugated moiety [58] reflecting fetal adrenal hypoplasia.

Dexamethasone treatment of the mother (n = 5) (8 mg dexamethasone 8–20 h before elective cesarean section) resulted in undetectable levels of the free moiety in all cases. However, the concentration of 17 OH-Preg sulfate was within the normal range in three and subnormal in two. The mean for this group was not significantly different from the normal controls [58].

4. Other Δ^5-C_{21} Steroids

Besides the data given in the previous chapter, no further studies on measurements of these steroids in human amniotic fluid have been published.

IV. Δ^4-C_{21} Steroids

1. Progesterone

a) Normal Pregnancies

The methods for the measurement of progesterone in amniotic fluid are compiled in Table 2. Throughout normal pregnancy, the concentration of progesterone declines according to Johansson and Jonasson [126] from 55.3 (13–16 weeks of gestation) to 26.4 μg/liter (37–40 weeks of gestation) and is in contrast to the rising maternal plasma concentration as shown in Fig. 1. Similar results were obtained by Younglai et al. [125] who reported a mean concentration of 61.9 μg/liter between the 11th and 15th week of gestation and a decrease to 29.5 μg/liter until the 36th to 40th week. The decrease of progesterone concentration in amniotic fluid was already demonstrated by Zander and Münstermann [61], measuring samples from the 1st trimester of

Table 2. Methods used for determination of progesterone in human amniotic fluid

Year of publication	Method	Ref.
1956	Spectrophotometry	61
1964	Spectrophotometry	122
1966	GLC	123
1967	Double isotope-derivative method	124
1968	GLC	57
1971	Competitive protein binding	125
1971	Competitive protein binding	126
1972	Competitive protein binding	127
1975	GLC	62
1976	RIA	128
1977	RIA	99
1977	RIA	86
1979	RIA	87
1979	RIA	129

Table 3. Progesterone in human amniotic fluid throughout normal gestation [129]

Weeks of gestation	n	Progesterone (μg/liter; mean ± SEM)
9–16	10	39.9 ± 5.6
38	2	19.9 ± 5.0
39	3	14.7 ± 4.2
40	9	16.6 ± 1.9
41	3	13.6 ± 6.2
42	6	14.5 ± 2.4

gestation until term. Our unpublished results [129] obtained by RIA confirm this as shown in Table 3. This was also confirmed by the data reported by Warne et al. [99], also indicating that differences according to the sex of the fetus are not present as shown in Table 4. These data have subsequently been confirmed (Table 5), [86, 87].

Table 4. Progesterone in human amniotic fluid throughout pregnancy according to the sex of the fetus [99]

Weeks of gestation	Progesterone (μg/liter; mean and range)				P[a]
	Male	n	Female	n	
9–<12	22 (15–49)	7	21 (7–41)	4	NS
12–<16	31 (10–55)	23	32 (10–133)	22	NS
16–<19	24 (7–60)	19	27 (13–47)	14	NS
28–<34	21 (17–30)	4	–	–	–
34– 40	6 (4–25)	11	15 (5–24)	9	0.04

[a] P, Statistical significance of sex differences

The decrease of progesterone in amniotic fluid during the course of pregnancy was found by Nagamani et al. [87] to be significant ($P < 0.05$).

The reason for the decline of this steroid in amniotic fluid throughout gestation is not clear. Since the concentration of most of the steroids in amniotic fluid are regulated by fetal urinary excretion, this could account for

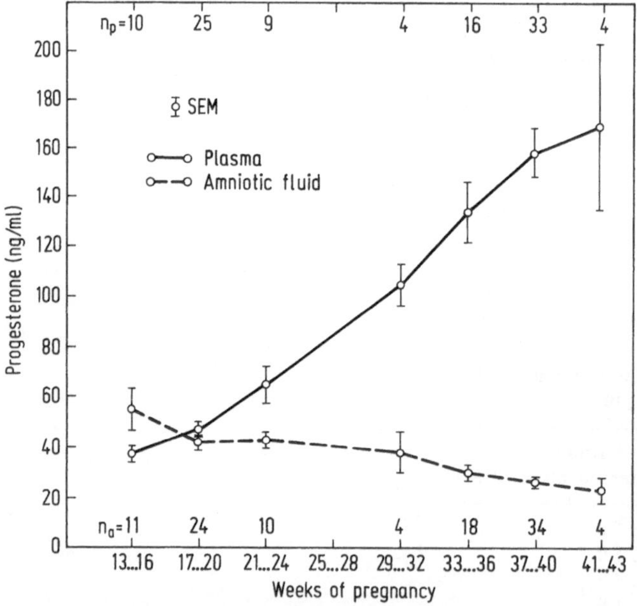

Fig. 1. Levels of progesterone in plasma and amniotic fluids from the same patients. The values are groupes in 4-week periods. n_p, number of plasma samples in each 4-week period; n_a, number of amniotic fluid samples in each 4-week period. (Johansson and Janasson 1971 [126])

Table 5. Progesterone in human amniotic fluid according to week of gestation and sex of the fetus

Weeks of gestation	Fetal sex	n	Progesterone (μg/liter; mean ± SEM)	Ref.
14–22	Male	66	55.0 ± 3.4	86
	Female	33	54.0 ± 4.5	
14–20	Male	–	34.7 ± 4.1	87
	Female	–	30.1 ± 4.0	
28–40	Male	–	14.1 ± 3.1	87
	Female	–	13.3 ± 2.1	

the changes of this unconjugated water-insoluble steroid in human amniotic fluid, which in turn can be influenced by protein binding in the fetal circulation during gestation, increased utilization, and metabolism by the maturing fetus. Direct transfer from the amniotic membranes and placenta also has to be considered since these structures contain a far greater concentration of this steroid [123, 130]. Taking the changes in total amniotic fluid volume into account, it was concluded that there is no decline of fetal progesterone in amniotic fluid as pregnancy progresses [99].

Similar results in the last trimester were obtained by Lurie et al. [123] with 39 μg/liter, Schindler and Siiteri [57] with 39.4 μg/liter, Ylikorkala et al. [131] with 40.6 ± 11.2 (SD) μg/liter, Friedrich et al. [62] with 50 μg/liter (range 47–60 μg/liter), and Harbert et al. [122] with 59 ± 7.5 (SD) μg/liter. Slightly higher values between the 36th and 38th week (n = 3) were reported by Wiest [124] with an average concentration of 124 μg/liter as well as by Zander and Münstermann [61] for the first half of pregnancy (n = 8) with 166 μg/liter.

b) Complicated Pregnancies

Progesterone in amniotic fluid was measured by Jonasson and Johansson in various abnormal conditions of pregnancy [132]. Their data are listed in Table 6.

Table 6. Progesterone in human amniotic fluid in complicated pregnancies [132]

Clinical condition	Progesterone (μg/liter; mean + SEM)					
	29–32 weeks of gestation	n	33–36 weeks of gestation	n	37–40 weeks of gestation	n
Rh group I	51.7	1	37.6 ± 3.3	14	29.7 ± 2.0	24
Rh group II	38.7 ± 8.6	3	32.5 ± 1.8	32	27.0 ± 0.9	28
Rh group III	42.0 ± 3.5	13	34.1 ± 2.3	22	31.6 ± 2.8	11
Rh group IV	39.9 ± 5.7	5	39.3 ± 3.1	9	39.6 ± 7.3	4
Hepatosis	24.7	1	25.5 ± 1.0	3	34.4 ± 4.8	6
Preeclampsia	40.0	1	35.5	1	39.3	1
Hydramnios	36.1	1	–	–	32.5	2

There is a tendency toward higher progesterone values in Rh isoimmunization of a mild to severe degree, which is not statistically significant.

In pregnancies with ultimate fetal death due to Rh isoimmunization, there is a rise particularly during the last two 4-week periods ($0.05 > P > 0.025$ and $0.01 > P > 0.005$, respectively). Three samples that reached values above 100 μg/liter were from pregnancies with hydropic fetuses that died of Rh isoimmunization within a few days after the sampling; however, meconium was present. All these data are in agreement with other findings that indicate increased placental activity in these conditions, leading to elevated values of placental enzymes and proteohormones and also to normal and even elevated steroid secretion. Even the fetal condition is disastrous as detailed elsewhere [133].

When progesterone in amniotic fluid was compared to the cord hemoglobin in cases with Rh isoimmunization, a tendency for higher progesterone values was associated with higher hemoglobin values [132]. This was statistically significant ($0.025 > P > 0.01$) if the hemoglobin value was 8.0 g/100 ml or lower. A significant correlation ($P < 0.001$) was also found between progesterone values in amniotic fluid and placental weight [132].

Also in hepatosis gravidarum, significantly ($0.05 > P > 0.025$) higher concentrations of progesterone were found between the 37th and 40th week [132]. Values obtained from pregnant women with preeclampsia, hydramnios, twin pregnancies, or diabetes were not different from the normal range [132]. Our data [129] are summarized in Table 7.

Table 7. Progesterone in human amniotic fluid in various clinical conditions [129]

Weeks of gestation	Progesterone (μg/liter; mean + SEM)							
	Edema	n	Rh incompatibility	n	Diabetes	n	Premature labor	n
28–31	33.6 ± 6.4	7	41.4 ± 5.8	10	–	–	39.6 ± 10.5	3
32–34	25.9 ± 2.4	8	28.8 ± 2.2	13	–	–	36.8 ± 7.5	4
35–37	16.7 ± 2.4	11	20.8 ± 2.7	13	53.4 ± 18.4	2	20.2 ± 2.3	14
38	17.3 ± 1.6	11	15.9 ± 1.5	4	21.7 ± 0.7	2	18.5 ± 5.5	3
39	18.0 ± 4.9	5	19.8 ± 1.0	2	24.3	1	15.6 ± 3.7	4
40	18.8 ± 1.4	11	–	–	–	–	–	–
41	17.8 ± 2.9	8	–	–	27.0 ± 0.7	2	28.9 ± 5.6	2
42	13.8 ± 3.2	4	–	–	–	–	–	–

The corresponding normal values are listed in Table 3. The values in diabetic pregnancies are higher. Slightly higher values are also noted for Rh incompatibility; however, a differentiation according to the severity of fetal involvement was not done. In a case with congenital adrenal hyperplasia of the fetus examined at 22 weeks of gestation, progesterone levels were indistinguishable from normal levels with values of 15, 15, and 20 ng/ml, respectively [87]. In a pregnancy with hydropic degeneration of the placenta, a very high concentration of 160 ng/ml of progesterone was found [87]. Maternal dexamethasone therapy did not change the progesterone concentration in amniotic fluid [134].

A unique finding was observed in pregnancies aborted with prostaglandin $F_{2\alpha}$ during the second trimester [128]. In contrast to the decrease of plasma progesterone after prostaglandin injection into maternal plasma, there was a steady and considerable increase in progesterone concentration in the amniotic fluid. The authors explained this by a decreased uterine blood flow accompanied by sustained amniotic resting pressure of more than 40 mmHg leading to an extravasation of placental and membrane progesterone into the amniotic fluid [128].

In two studies, the influence of betamethasone or dexamethasone administration to the mother for fetal lung maturation on amniotic fluid progesterone values was investigated in patients at risk [131, 135]. The results obtained are shown in Table 8. No significant differences were found.

Table 8. Progesterone in human amniotic fluid before and after betamethasone treatment

	n	Progesterone (μg/liter; mean + SEM)		Ref.
		Amniocentesis I	Amniocentesis II	
Betamethasone group	8	33.7 ± 5.1	37.3 ± 5.1	135
Control group	5	27.2 ± 4.2	26.9 ± 4.9	
Dexamethasone group	10	40.6 ± 11.2	41.6 ± 16.3	131

2. 16α-Hydroxyprogesterone

Except for the quantitation during the isolation and identification procedures [62], no further measurements of this steroid in human amniotic fluid have been reported. Eight determinations in normal amniotic fluid at term resulted in a mean concentration of 130 μg/liter with a range of 114–147 μg/liter [62].

3. 17α-Hydroxyprogesterone

This steroid was measured by radioimmunoassay by Tulchinsky and Simmer [136]. A concentration of 0.6 ± 0.1 (SEM) μg/liter was found in midpregnancy (n = 8) and 1.1 ± 0.3 (SEM) μg/liter at term (n = 5) [63]. In 13 amniotic fluid samples from high-risk pregnancies between the 24th and 38th week of gestation, Frasier et al. [63] measured the mean amniotic fluid concentration of this steroid to be 0.7 ± 0.05 (SEM) μg/liter with a range between 0.4 and 1.0 μg/liter. A sex difference could not be detected, and a change with increasing gestation was not seen. More recently, Warne et al. [99] noted that the concentration of this steroid in amniotic fluid between the 12th and 18th week of gestation was significantly higher than in late pregnancy. A sex difference was not observed (Table 9).

Taking all the data from the 9th to 19th week of gestation, however, a significant difference ($P < 0.02$) between female [1.09 ± 0.07 (SEM) μg/liter, n = 35] and male fetuses [0.85 ± 0.07 (SEM) μg/liter, n = 33] evolved. This could be due to a sex difference in fetal 17α-hydroxylation of progesterone or a difference in placental synthesis of 17α-hydroxyprogesterone from 17α-hydroxy-

Table 9. 17α-Hydroxyprogesterone in human amniotic fluid according to fetal age and sex [99]

Weeks of gestation	17α-Hydroxyprogesterone (μg/liter; mean and range)				P[a]
	Male	n	Female	n	
9–<12	0.44 (0.22–0.52)	4	0.74 (40–146)	3	NS
12–<16	0.88 (0.47–1.64)	17	0.97 (0.56–1.95)	18	NS
16–<19	0.92 (0.45–1.60)	12	0.94 (0.86–2.50)	14	NS
28–<34	0.47 (0.40–1.09)	4	–	–	–
34– 40	0.51 (0.22–0.78)	6	0.46 (0.25–0.65)	10	NS

[a] P, Significance of sex differences

pregnenolone. Indeed, an umbilical arteriovenous difference in progesterone concentration at term has been reported [137]. Others could not detect sex differences [87, 121, 136].

So far, only a few reports have been published on 17α-hydroxyprogesterone in amniotic fluid from pregnancies subsequently shown to have carried a fetus affected with congenital adrenal hyperplasia due to 21-hydroxylase deficiency [63, 87, 121, 136, 138]. The mean concentration in such a pregnancy was 1.88 ± 0.32 (SEM) μg/liter with a range of 1.10–2.95 μg/liter in six determinations [136]. These values, however, overlap with the values reported by Warne et al. [99] for normal pregnancies. More recently, Nagamani et al. [138] found in normal pregnancies a concentration range of 0.25–2.66 μg/liter resulting in a mean value of 1.33 ± 0.07 (SEM) μg/liter. Fetal sex-dependent differences were not detected. The mean level of 1.57 ± 0.08 μg/liter during 14–24 weeks of gestation was significantly higher than the mean level of 0.79 ± 0.06 μg/liter obtained during late pregnancy ($P < 0.001$).

The same authors have published further data [87] showing a decrease from 1.62 ± 0.15 to 0.87 ± 0.15 ng/ml from 14 to 20 weeks of gestation in males and from 1.51 ± 0.1 to 0.69 ± 0.08 ng/ml in females.

In affected pregnancies, the level of 17α-hydroxyprogesterone was higher during all stages of pregnancy (8.23 at 14 weeks, 20.68 at 22 weeks, 2.93 at

Table 10. 17α-Hydroxyprogesterone in human amniotic fluid between 15 and 20 weeks of gestation in normal pregnancy (Wurster et al., unpublished results)

Weeks of gestation	17α-Hydroxyprogesterone (ng/ml; mean ± SD)					
	Male	n	Female	n	Male + Female	n
15	–	–	4.19 ± 1.48	2	–	–
16	3.49 ± 0.78	14	4.07 ± 1.12	12	3.76 ± 0.98	26
17	3.43 ± 0.56	33	3.01 ± 0.56	20	3.27 ± 0.59	53
18	3.46 ± 0.93	26	3.05 ± 0.71	18	3.30 ± 0.86	44
19	3.07 ± 0.92	7	3.18 ± 0.65	11	3.14 ± 0.74	18
20	2.87 ± 0.54	4	3.14 ± 0.75	7	3.04 ± 0.67	11
15–20	–	–	–	–	3.34 ± 0.80	152

28 weeks, and 3.67 μg/liter at 34 weeks). Similar to the control values, the 17α-hydroxyprogesterone levels were higher before 24 weeks compared to the level after 24 weeks [87, 138]. Milunsky and Tulchinsky [121] detected retrospectively at 16 weeks of gestation a sevenfold increase in concentration of 17α-hydroxyprogesterone over the mean level of normal patients at the same stage of gestation, which is well above the 95% confidence limits for normal patients. Since prenatal diagnostic attempts have expanded, larger series of data will become available. Results of such a study are listed in Table 10. It is obvious that there is a gradual decrease in the concentration of 17 OH-Prog as gestation advances. In pregnancies with heterozygous fetuses, 17 OH-Prog values in amniotic fluid range between 2.64 and 2.97 ng/ml

Table 11. Methods used for the determination of cortisol in human amniotic fluid

Year of publication	Method	Ref.
1954	Tetrazolium blue	64
1955	Tetrazolium blue	139
1960	NaOH fluorescence	65
1963	Triphenyl tetrazolium Chloridereaction	56
1971	Competitive proteinbinding	66
1971	Double isotope-derivative technique	67
1973	Competitive proteinbinding	140
1974	Competitive proteinbinding	141
1975	Competitive proteinbinding	142
1975	RIA	143
1975	Radiotransinassay	144
1975	Competitive proteinbinding	145
1975	Radiotransinassay	146
1975	RIA	147
1975	Competitive proteinbinding	148
1976	Competitive proteinbinding	149
1976	Competitive proteinbinding	150
1976	High-speed liquid chromatography	151
1976	RIA	152
1977	Radiotransinassay	153
1977	Competitive proteinbinding	154
1977	Competitive proteinbinding	155
1977	Radiotransinassay	152
1977	RIA	156
1977	Competitive proteinbinding	157
1977	RIA	158
1977	RIA	71
1978	Competitive proteinbinding	159
1978	RIA	160
1978	RIA	70
1979	RIA	129
1979	RIA	161
1979	RIA	134
1980	RIA	70

at 17–18 weeks of gestation. In a pregnancy with a homozygously affected fetus, the value was about ten times higher, i. e., 22 ng/ml (Wurster et al., unpublished results).

4. Cortisol

Quite a number of methods have been developed for the measurement of cortisol in amniotic fluid. A summary is given in Table 11.

a) Normal Pregnancies

According to the first report, cortisol did not appear to be present in normal amniotic fluid [64]. Later, it was detected in normal amniotic fluid and reported to be present as the free form in a concentration of 26 ± 3.2 (SEM) μg/liter [65]. While Nicholas et al. [56] concluded that cortisol is found in the free and glucuronide fraction in some amniotic fluid specimens (Table 12), others could detect this steroid only in the free and sulfate fraction [66, 67], resulting in a cortisol/cortisol sulfate ratio of 0.55 in amniotic fluid compared to umbilical cord plasma (2.4) and maternal plasma (127.0) [67]. In ten samples, a concentration of cortisol sulfate of 34.1 ± 11.6 (SD) μg/liter was found [66]. Comparing the values of the free and sulfoconjugated forms, values of 18 versus 30 μg/liter [66] and 20 versus 36 μg/liter [67] have been reported.

Table 12. Free and conjugated cortisol in normal human amniotic fluid according to Nicholas et al. [56]

Amniotic fluid (ml)	Cortisol (μg/liter)	
	Free	Conjugated
275	10.0	10.0
360	20.0	20.0
660	0.0	0.0
857	0.0	0.0
3 800 (trias)	10.0	10.0
400	0.0	0.0

The data obtained for cortisol have to be considered in relation to the various cortisol moieties that have been determined and in part exhibit considerable quantitative differences. Results on free and total cortisol in amniotic fluid are compiled in Tables 13 and 14. The differences in free and total cortisol in amniotic fluid have recently been clearly demonstrated [159].

There are differences in the absolute values depending on the type of method used, particularly toward term as shown in Table 14. A sharp increase prior to delivery is obvious from the data of Jolivet [141, 165]. The cortisol level 10–30 days prior to birth was 23.0 ± 5.3 (SD) μg/liter, 1–5 days prior it was 33.2 ± 7.4 (SD) μg/liter, and on the day of parturition it was 44.3 ± 13.8 (SD) μg/liter for term deliveries. In premature deliveries, similar changes occurred at a lower level with 18.3 ± 5.1 (SD), 30.8 ± 9.3, and 35.6 ± 7.9 (SD) μg/liter respectively [141].

Comparison of amniotic fluid cortisol levels in cases with premature labor and pregnancies of the same gestational age without labor demonstrates higher amniotic fluid cortisol levels in pregnancies with premature labor: 32.7 versus 17.0 ng/ml [165].

Generally, there is a change of concentration as pregnancy progresses toward term [70, 71, 134, 144, 150, 153, 161, 164, 166]. According to Murphy et al. [144], the concentration of free cortisol in amniotic fluid gradually increases during gestation with a rapid rise at 38–40 weeks [144] as demonstrated in Fig. 2. There was an initial rise during the 2nd trimester followed by a plateau with a tendency to a fall at 33–35 weeks and a sharp increase 1–2 weeks before delivery with a peak at 40 weeks. The difference between the mean level at 38–40 weeks and over, 34–37 weeks, 20–30 weeks, and 8–17 weeks was highly significant ($P < 0.001$). At least for the last trimester a similar tendency was found by others [147] although the absolute values were different as shown in Table 15.

Table 13. Free cortisol in human amniotic fluid

Weeks of gestation	n	Free cortisol (µg/liter; mean ± SEM)	Method	Ref.
At term	10	26 ±3.2[a]	Fluorometry	65
Near term	23	17.8 ± 6.7[a]	Competitive protein binding	142
<36	43	25.2 ± 1.4	RIA	162
>36	17	33.4 ± 2.6	RIA	
13–24	9	8.9	RIA	158
37–38	6	13.8		
39–40	9	19.5		
At the onset of labor	5	25.6 ± 3.5	RIA	144
<20	26	8.6 ± 0.8	Competitive protein binding	150
20–25	16	11.4 ± 1.2		
30–40	36	19.8 ± 1.5		
>40	5	22.9 ± 2.8		
>30	76	20.2 ± 1.3	Competitive protein binding	163
35–40	98	27	RIA	153
At term	19	69.4 ± 7.4	RIA	164
9–20	69	6.5	RIA	70a
28–37	21	13.9		
11–16	11	3.9 ± 0.6	RIA	271
17–22	11	4.7 ± 0.9		
25–30	4	9.4 ± 1.7		
36–40 (no labor)	7	18.0 ± 3.0		
36–40 (spontaneous labor)	5	28.5 ± 8.3		

[a] Mean ± SD

Table 14. Total cortisol in human amniotic fluid

Weeks of gestation	n	Total cortisol (μg/liter)	Method	Ref.
At term	12	53 ± 26	Competitive protein binding	140[a]
<20		30 ± 2	RIA	143[b]
20–24		31.8 ± 1.5		
35–40		72.4 ± 3.8		
>40		139 ± 12		
<32	13	139 ± 124	RIA	147[a]
33–34	8	103 ± 32		
35–36	17	144 ± 117		
33–40	45	202 ± 95		
41–42	12	290 ± 78		
>42	3	204 ± 34		
9–16	10	33.4 ± 4.9	RIA	129[b]
38	2	242.9 ± 110.6		
39	3	187.8 ± 35.7		
40	8	183.6 ± 28.5		
41	3	168.7 ± 28.6		
42	6	203.6 ± 26.8		
28	10	34.1 ± 13.3	RIA	161[a]
31	9	32.9 ± 5.2		
34	25	39.2 ± 13.8		
37	41	48.8 ± 13.8		
40	28	60.1 ± 20.2		
41	6	65.7 ± 24.1		
34–42	58	34.5 ± 17.5	RIA	134[a]

[a] All values = Mean ± SD
[b] All values = Mean ± SEM

Rising concentrations were obtained for total cortisol [143] as demonstrated in Fig. 3 and also reported by others [134, 147, 151, 159, 160, 161]. The importance of corticosteroids for initiation of labor and delivery was extensively studied by Liggins et al. [167], and the influence of corticoids on human fetal lung maturation was demonstrated [168].

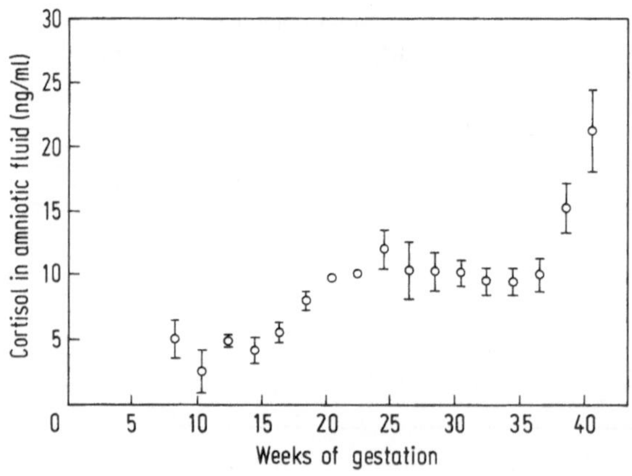

Fig. 2. Mean cortisol level in amniotic fluid at various gestational ages prior to the onset of labor. The *bars* show SEM. (Murphy et al. 1975 [144])

Table 15. Cortisol concentration in human amniotic fluid according to Sivakumaran et al. [147]

Weeks of gestation	n	Cortisol (μg/liter; mean ± SD)
32	13	139 ± 124
33–34	8	103 ± 32
35–36	17	144 ± 117
37–40	45	202 ± 95
41–42	12	290 ± 78
42	3	204 ± 34

Indeed, cortisol levels in umbilical cord blood in neonates who subsequently developed hyaline membrane disease were shown to be lower than those in normal newborns of comparable age [169]. Lecithin and sphingomyelin as well as other substances reflect human fetal lung maturation [170, 171]. Therefore, several studies have been undertaken to evaluate cortisol levels in amniotic fluid and fetal lung function. Amniotic fluid cortisol levels and lecithin/sphingomyelin (L/S) ratios were determined simultaneously in 43 amniotic fluid samples obtained from normal patients at various stages of gestation [143]. Total cortisol levels higher than 60 μg/liter (n = 26) were associated in 23 cases with lecithin/sphingomyelin ratios higher than 2.0, in three cases with ratios between 1.5 and 2.0. In none of the newborns of 16 patients of this group delivered within 48 h of the time the amniotic fluid was obtained did fetal respiratory distress develop. At a level between 40 and 60 μg/liter (n = 5), the L/S ratio was in one higher than 2.0, in three cases between 1.5 and 2.0, and in one case lower than 1.5. Two of these were delivered within 48 h and developed mild respiratory distress syndrome (RDS). In 12 cases the umbilical cord levels were below 40 μg/liter; the L/S ratio was below 1.5. No delivery occurred within 48 h. The association between cortisol values and the lecithin/sphingomyelin ratios was highly significant ($P < 0.001$).

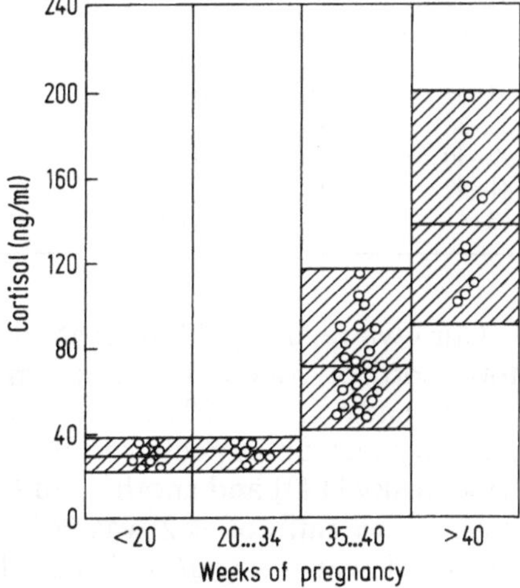

Fig. 3. Total cortisol concentration in amniotic fluid at various stages of pregnancy. The *middle line* in each *bar* represents the mean value for the group; the *shaded areas* represent the skewed 95% confidence limits of normal values. (Fencl and Tulchinsky 1975 [143])

Similar results were obtained by others using identical grouping of the L/S ratio results [150]. In uncomplicated pregnancies, the correlation was highly significant ($P < 0.001$). Considering only data after 30 weeks of gestation, a similar significance was obtained ($P < 0.005$). Sequential analysis demonstrates that a cortisol rise paralleled the maturation of the L/S ration [150], while in another report this was not as obvious [147]. Direct correlation with lecithin also demonstrated significance [172].

Smith et al. [152] found a lower cortisol level in human amniotic fluid in respiratory distress syndrome [19.2 ± 7.2 (SD) versus 26.1 ± 9.4 (SD) μg/liter, $P < 0.02$]. Looking at infants below 32 weeks of gestation, similar results were observed in this subgroup [18.2 ± 12.9 (SD) versus 29.7 ± 4.7 (SD) μg/liter, $P < 0.05$]. In the group at or above 32 weeks, significant differences were no longer observed [20.2 ± 7.5 (SD) versus 25.6 ± 9.8 (SD) μg/liter].

Since the incidence of respiratory distress in premature infants of patients whose labor commences after rupture of the membranes is lower [173], a comparison was carried out with patients whose labor had begun with contractions or bleeding [152]. No significant difference in amniotic fluid cortisol levels was found [24.8 ± 9.9 (SD) versus 22.8 ± 11.3 (SD) μg/liter]. Johnson and Hensleigh [157] found, however, that among 34 patients delivering within 72 h of cortisol measurement a range from 10 to 309 μg/liter was present. Applying the critical cortisol level of 60 μg/liter of amniotic fluid suggested by Fencl and Tulchinsky [143] for predicting lung maturity, 26 specimens with a lower level had L/S ratios above 2.0. Half of the cases tested within 72 h of delivery had low amniotic fluid cortisol levels, but some showed subsequent evidence of RDS [157].

A wide scatter of the cortisol and L/S ratio results are obvious from the data by Sivakumaran et al. [147], which correlate with the data grouped according to weeks of gestation as shown in Table 16.

Table 16. Human amniotic fluid cortisol concentration and L/S ratio according to weeks of gestation [147]

Weeks of gestation	n	Cortisol (μg/liter; mean ± SD)	L/S ratio (Mean ± SD)
32	13	139 ± 124	1.8 ± 2.3
33–34	8	103 ± 32	1.4 ± 1.0
35–36	17	144 ± 117	2.3 ± 2.1
37–40	45	202 ± 95	2.9 ± 2.2
41–42	12	250 ± 78	3.9 ± 2.0
42	3	204 ± 34	3.0 ± 1.1

Our own results [129] indicate that between 35 and 38 weeks of gestation the total cortisol concentration in amniotic fluid and L/S ratio $\leqq$ 3.0 correlated significantly ($P < 0.001$). At the level of more than 100 ng/ml cortisol, lung maturity can be expected in 96%. This is comparable to data by Fencl and Tulchinsky [143] and another study [166]. The incidence of respiratory distress with a L/S ratio of $\geqq 2$ was 26% if the cortisol was < 43 ng/ml and 2.9% if the level was $\geqq$ 43 ng/ml. This difference was significant ($P < 0.05$). Doran

Table 17. Predictive value and efficiency of methods for determination of fetal lung maturity [161]

Methods and cortisol value	Predictive value of immature results	Predictive value of mature results	Efficiency
L/S ratio ≧ 3	11%	98%	82%
Total cortisol ≧ 30 ng/ml	33	97	92
Lipid positive cells ≧ 10%	100	98	98
Palmitic acid ≧ 9 mg/liter	8	97	76
P/S ratio[a] ≧ 3.7	5	97	62
Creatinine ≧ 1.8 mg%	9	97	74

[a] P/S, palmitic/stearic ratio

et al. [161] calculated the predictive value of immature (positive) results, the predictive value of mature (negative) results, and the efficiency of various methods for evaluating lung maturity. The data are summarized in Table 17.

Mean levels of palmitic acid concentration, palmitic/stearic ratio, and cortisol showed an increase during the last part of pregnancy. The correlation of cortisol with palmitic acid (n = 92) considered individually was weak (r = 0.48, $P < 0.001$). A slightly higher correlation was found between cortisol and the palmitic/stearic ratio (r = 0.65, $P < 0.001$). Taking only samples after 28 weeks of gestation, the correlation coefficient dropped to 0.28 ($P < 0.05$ and 0.55, $P < 0.001$, respectively). Excluding pathologic pregnancies and samples before 28 weeks and dividing according to high (> 20 μg/liter) versus low (< 15 μg/liter) cortisol levels and mature versus immature palmitic acid concentrations, five of six samples with low cortisol had immature palmitic acid concentrations, whereas 21 of 24 with high cortisol had mature palmitic acid levels [153]. Similar results were obtained for the palmitic/stearic ratios. Despite a significant χ^2 value ($P < 0.005$), almost one-third of the samples with high palmitic acid concentration and palmitic/stearic ratios had low cortisol levels [153]. Similar results were found by others [70]. A significant increase in cortisol at 28–39 weeks of gestation preceded the greatest increase in palmitic acid [70].

Failure to demonstrate correlations between palmitic acid and cortisol in amniotic fluid was reported by Bichler and Geir [174].

Table 18. Human amniotic fluid cortisol levels in term and premature deliveries [140]

	Cortisol (μg/liter; mean ± SD)			
	Term deliveries	n	Premature deliveries	n
Spontaneous labor	53 ± 2.6	16	35 ± 1.0	6
Induced labor	26 ± 6.0	4	–	–
Cesarean section	24 ± 0.8	9	23	3

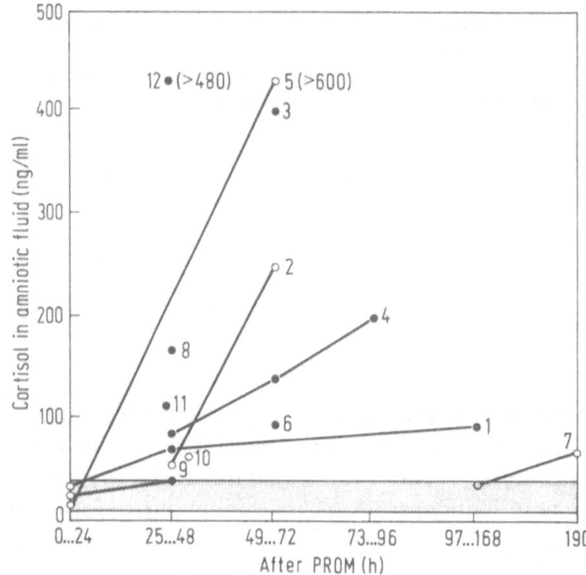

Fig. 4. Cortisol concentration in amniotic fluid following premature rupture of membranes (PROM) of four patients (Nos. *2, 5, 7,* and *10*) at 24–26 weeks of gestation (○) and eight patients at 30–34 weeks of gestation (●). The *shaded area* represents amniotic fluid concentration of patients at 21–34 weeks of gestation with premature rupture of membranes of less than 3 h duration. (From Cohen, Wayne, Fencl, Montserrat deM., and Tulchinsky, Dan: Amniotic fluid cortisol after premature rupture of membranes, J. Pediatr. 88:1007–1009, 1976 [173a])

Divergent results have been reported on amniotic fluid cortisol levels and labor. While Pokoly [140] found significant differences as listed in Table 18, others could not detect such differences [149, 162].

More recently, a rise in amniotic fluid cortisol levels in labor was reported [164].

Rupture of the membranes, a factor in fetal lung maturation [173], was shown to be associated with a rise in amniotic fluid cortisol levels 24 h after rupture as shown in Fig. 4. [173a] A similar finding in one case was reported by Gewolb et al. [163]. This could reflect increased cortisol biosynthesis, but may also be related to changes in amniotic fluid volume. Recently, it was suggested that the amniotic fluid cortisol and maternal serum cortisol ratio be considered an indicator for fetal lung maturity [134].

b) Complicated Pregnancies

In anencephaly, Fencl et al. [175] found amniotic fluid values below the 95% confidence limit of normal pregnancies. Data of five other reports [140, 144, 153, 163, 176] did not reveal such differences. In a case of congenital fetal adrenal hypoplasia, the amniotic fluid cortisol level was low [177].

In Rh isoimmunization, there is no difference compared to normal values except for severe involvement. In these cases the levels are high [144]. The data published by Gewolb et al. [163] indicate higher levels in Rh isoimmunization between 20 and 25 weeks of gestation ($P < 0.05$) and lower levels after 30 weeks of gestation ($P < 0.05$). This finding applies also to our own unpublished data listed in Table 19.

Table 19. Human amniotic fluid cortisol levels in Rh isoimmunization [129]

Weeks of gestation	n	Cortisol (μg/liter; mean ± SEM)
28–31	9	65.7 ± 2.4
32–34	13	72.0 ± 5.6
35–37	15	79.5 ± 6.0
38	4	104.9 ± 8.5
39	2	155.1 ± 18.2

In pregnancies involving high blood pressure or toxemia, Cope et al. [139] reported a mean concentration of 16 μg/liter (n = 6). Higher than normal values were found by others [163]. The difference was not marked in those patients with immature L/S ratios [21.4 ± 2.9 versus 15.4 ± 1.4 (SD) μg/liter, $P < 0.05$]. Our own data are listed in Table 20.

Table 20. Human amniotic fluid cortisol levels in toxemia [129]

Weeks of gestation	n	Cortisol (μg/liter; mean ± SEM)
29	1	75.7
32	1	120.3
34	1	75.5
39	3	206.3 ± 43.0
40	1	189.4
41	4	198.5 ± 25.1

First it was thought that cortisol is only present in amniotic fluid from pregnancies of diabetics [64]. Further studies, however, established similar levels in normal and diabetic pregnancies [56, 65]. Gewolb et al. [173] found significantly higher levels in samples of pregnancies over 30 weeks [15.7 ± 1.2 (SD) versus 20.2 ± 1.3 (SD) μg/liter, $P < 0.02$]. It is noteworthy that according to L/S ratios those with values < 2 had significantly lower cortisol levels than normal 17.5 ± 1.5 (SD) μg/liter. The rise of the cortisol level in amniotic fluid usually seen after 35 weeks of gestation was found to be delayed or absent in patients with diabetes [166]. Lower values were also demonstrated by Goldkrand [164] and Pschera et al. [423]. In both studies the differences were not significant. The severity of the diabetic disease did not affect the cortisol levels in amniotic fluid and there was no correlation between total cortisol concentration and L/S-ration in amniotic fluid [423].

In a pregnancy with placental sulfatase deficiency, the cortisol levels were similar to normal controls, demonstrating that the fetal adrenal is not involved in this condition [178]. In a pregnancy with a cephalothoracopagus, the cortisol concentration in amniotic fluid was 212 μg/liter at 28 weeks of gestation [179].

Recent knowledge on fetal lung maturation [168, 171] has introduced the application of potent synthetic corticoids to enhance fetal lung maturation and to prevent the respiratory distress syndrome of the newborn [169]. Besides the well-known changes in maternal urinary estriol excretion [148, 171] and corresponding precursors [179a], such treatment leads to changes of the cortisol concentration in amniotic fluid. This was first demonstrated by Ohrlander et al. [148] (see Fig. 5). More detailed data (Table 21) were given later [162].

Table 21. Changes of cortisol concentration in human amniotic fluid under treatment with betamethasone [162]

Days between start of study and delivery	Cortisol (μg/liter: mean ± SEM)				
	Amniocentesis I	Amniocentesis II	P[a]	Delivery	P[a]
Betamethasone treated					
≦7 days 4.0 ± 1.1	29.4 ± 8.7 (n = 3)	6.7 ± 1.7 (n = 3)	NS	9.3 ± 2.4 (n = 4)	NS
8–21 days 15.0 ± 1.5	25.6 ± 3.8 (n = 4)	5.4 ± 0.6 (n = 5)	<0.01	30.7 ± 13.0 (n = 5)	NS
>21 days 43.9 ± 3.2	22.8 ± 1.5 (n = 11)	5.0 ± 0.5 (n = 11)	<0.001	31.1 ± 2.6 (n = 10)	<0.05
Total 28.7 ± 3.9	24.5 ± 1.8 (n = 18)	5.4 ± 0.4 (n = 19)	<0.001	26.4 ± 4.0 (n = 19)	NS
Controls 29.7 ± 4.3	28.2 ± 2.9 (n = 17)	25.6 ± 2.2 (n = 14)	NS	38.1 ± 2.9 (n = 12)	<0.05

[a] P, Statistical evaluation

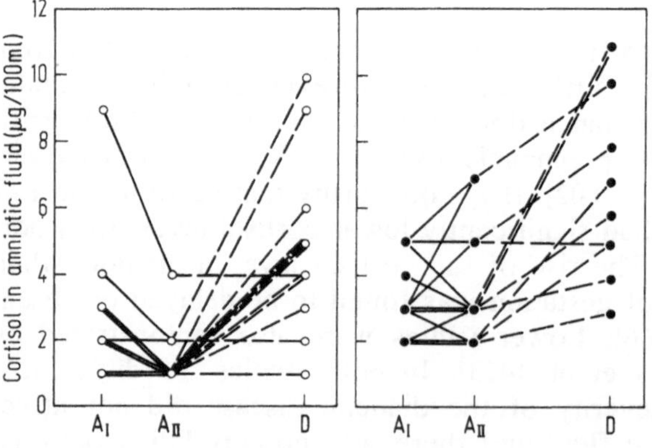

Fig. 5. Cortisol concentration in amniotic fluid of 15 women with betamethasone treatment *(left, open symbols)* and of 12 control subjects *(right, solid symbols)*. *Solid* and *dashed lines* unite values from the same woman. A_I and A_{II} denote amniocentesis 4 days apart; *D* indicates delivery. Betamethasone, 12 mg daily for 3 days, was given to women in left graph between A_I and A_{II}. (Ohrlander et al. 1975 [148])

As demonstrated in Table 20, the cortisol concentration in amniotic fluid decreases significantly after betamethasone treatment and again reaches nearly normal levels at the time of delivery if the interval is longer than 7 days after drug administration. Such a cortisol reduction was also reported by others [155, 180] as shown in Table 22.

Table 22. Effect of antepartum betamethasone on cortisol in human amniotic fluid in pregnancies with delivery before 37 weeks gestation [155]

	n	Cortisol (μg/liter)		P[a]
		Mean ± SEM	Range	
Untreated	7	18.5 ±2.1	13.0 ± 28.2	<0.001
Treated	5	9.3 ± 1.9	3.1 – 14.9	

[a] P, Statistical evaluation

Cortisol levels in amniotic fluid were also studied before and after prostaglandin administration [154, 156]. In pregnancies at 16–23 weeks of gestation, there was a significant increase in the concentration of cortisol in amniotic fluid following intra-amniotic injection of PGE_2, while such a change was not seen with $PGF_{2\alpha}$ [156]. The percentage change 4 h after injection of PGE_2 was 156 ± 22% (mean ± SEM) in contrast to PGF_2 (102 ± 9%, $P < 0.01$). In the

Table 23. Changes of cortisol concentration in amniotic fluid following intra-amniotic $PGF_{2\alpha}$ [154]

	Cortisol (μg/liter)				
	0 h	3 h	6 h	9 h	12 h
Case No. 1	27	62	105	81	–
2	32	27	53	40	47
3	26	15	68	–	–
4	34	39	65	91	63
5	30	42	44	–	–
6	18	46	64	–	–
7	59	65	98	83	90
8	28	23	75	137	114
9	32	25	44	–	–
10	73	65	95	–	–
11	96	122	183	186	–
12	91	118	89	–	–
13	56	41	55	–	–
14	56	68	68	89	83
Mean ± SD	47 ± 25.2	54 ± 32.7	79 ± 35.7	102.4 ± 46.6	79 ± 25.7
P[a]	–	NS	<0.001	<0.01	<0.02

[a] P, Statistical evaluation

PGE_2-treated group there was a gradual decrease in the concentration of cortisol in amniotic fluid after 4 h. In contrast, Koren et al. [154] reported an increase in the level of cortisol in amniotic fluid in response to $PGF_{2\alpha}$ injection. The time sequence is demonstrated in Table 23. However, at 3 h oxytocin infusion was started at a rate of 50 mU/min. [154].

A marked increase was noticed during oxytocin infusion (25 and 23 μg/liter) in the second and third 3-h periods, respectively. Before, the increase was only 7 μg/liter. Since cortisol in amniotic fluid seems to be mainly fetal in origin [154, 162], the rise could be due to fetal reaction toward augmentation of uterine contractions by oxytocin [154]. Failure to demonstrate changes in the cortisol level in amniotic fluid after $PGF_{2\alpha}$ could also be due to the differences in the amounts used [154, 156].

Some data have been published on correlations of cortisol levels in amniotic fluid with maternal and fetal levels. Early in pregnancy (16–23 weeks), no significant correlation between the cortisol concentration in paired samples of amniotic fluid and maternal plasma taken before and after prostaglandin administration was found [156]. A weak correlation ($r = 0.31$, $P = 0.05$) was found by Murphy et al. [144]; Tuimala et al. [149] described a correlation coefficient of $r = 0.41$, $P < 0.01$ during labor. The correlation was better in the latent phase ($r = 0.56$, $P < 0.01$) than in the active phase of the first stage of labor ($r = 0.28$, $P < 0.1$). On the average, better correlations were reported for amniotic fluid and cord blood levels. In the study by Pokoly [140], a weak correlation led to the conclusion that cortisol levels in amniotic fluid preclude estimation of cortisol concentration in fetal blood [140]. In another study [144], the correlation was good ($r = 0.69$, $P < 0.01$).

5. 6β-Hydroxycortisol and 6β,20β-Dihydroxycortisol

Only limited data are available regarding these steroids [108, 181]. The results in Table 24 in normal amniotic fluid during the 3rd trimester were obtained by Lambert and Pennington [181]. Drafta et al. [108] used the same method and reported the following results as compiled in Table 25.

In pregnancy complications such as diabetes, Rh isoimmunization, hydramnios, and anencephaly, lower values were reported as summarized in Table 26.

While 6β-hydroxycortisol was significantly decreased when compared

Table 24. 6β-Hydroxycortisol and 6β, 20β-dihydroxycortisol in normal human amniotic fluid during the 3rd trimester [181]

	6β-Hydroxycortisol (μg/liter)	6β, 20β-Dihydroxycortisol (μg/liter)
Case No. 1	23	4.0
2	50	6.0
3	54	7,0
4	35	3.0
5	45	0.0
6	54	28.0
Mean	43	8.0

Table 25. 6β-Hydroxycortisol and 6β, 20β-dihydroxycortisol in normal human amniotic fluid [108]

	6β-Hydroxycortisol (μg/liter)	6β, 20β-Dihydroxycortisol (μg/liter)
Case No. 1	150	150
2	100	60
3	100	60
4	60	60
5	20	60
6	160	80
7	80	80
8	66	80
9	110	100
10	50	50
11	80	40
12	50	70
13	20	120
14	100	100
15	50	120
16	70	160
17	20	65
18	20	–
Mean ± SEM	72.5 ± 4.2	76.4 ± 2.7

Table 26. Concentration of 6β-hydroxycortisol and 6β, 20β-dihydroxycortisol in human amniotic fluid in pathologic conditions of pregnancy [181]

	Diabetes	Rh isoimmunization	Hydramnios
	6β-Hydroxycortisol (μg/liter)		
Case No. 1	0.0	30.0	1.0
2	13.0	16.0	24.0
3	12.0	3.0	38.0
4	1.0	18.0	27.0
5	26.0	11.0	14.0
Mean	10.0	16.0	21.0
	6β, 20β-Dihydroxycortisol (μg/liter)		
Case No. 1	0.0	6.0	0.0
2	0.0	0.0	13.0
3	18.0	0.0	0.0
4	2.0	0.0	0.0
5	10.0	3.0	0.0
Mean	6.0	2.0	2.0

to the normal values (except in hydramnios), there was no significant difference for 6β, 20β-dihydroxycortisol levels [181]. The results reported for anencephaly are listed in Table 27 and demonstrate lower values for both steroids.

Table 27. 6β-Hydroxycortisol and 6β, 20β-dihydroxycortisol levels (μg/liter) in human amniotic fluid in anencephaly [108, 181]

	6β-Hydroxycortisol	6β, 20β-Dihydroxycortisol	Ref.
Case No. 1	1.0	0.0	181
2	0.0	0.0	
3	12.0	0.0	
4	18.0	3.0	
Mean	8.0	0.75	
Case No. 1	0.1	0.0	108

6. Cortisone

Several studies have been concerned with the measurement of cortisone in amniotic fluid. In normal pregnancies at term, Schweitzer et al. [66] measured cortisone sulfate in ten samples with a mean concentration of 26.5 ± 14.3 μg/liter (mean ± SD). From a pool, 11.0 μg of the free and 31.0 μl of sulfate moiety were found [66]. Before, the free moiety and the conjugated form were found in a concentration of 5.8 μg/liter each [56]. Recently, in 9 normal pregnancies at term free cortisone was found in a concentration of 9.0 ± 1.1 μg/liter (mean ± SEM) and cortisone sulfate in a concentration of 23.1 ± 6.1 μg/liter [424].

Due to the limited number of values no definite conclusions could be drawn regarding diabetes and toxemia [56]. Baird and Bush [65] did not detect differences between cortisone concentrations in amniotic fluid from normal and diabetic pregnancies (Table 28).

Studying premature deliveries, it was noticed that before 32 weeks of gestation the cortisone values were slightly higher when RDS developed in the infants (18.3 ± 9.2 versus 13.0 ± 2.4 μg/liter; *P*, NS) [152]. In the cases at or above 32 weeks of gestation, cortisone levels were not revealing (14.2 ± 4.0 versus 13.9 ± 3.9 μg/liter; *P*, NS).

Table 28. Cortisone level in human amniotic fluid in normal and diabetic pregnancies

	Cortisone (μg/liter)	
	Normal	Diabetes
Case No. 1	15.0	19.0
2	10.0	10.0
3	20.0	13.0
4	13.0	10.0
5	18.0	18.0
6	5.0	–
7	12.5	–
8	7.5	–
9	15.0	–
10	14.0	–
Mean ± SEM	13.0 ± 1.4	14.0 ± 1.9

At commencement of labor with ruptured membranes in comparison to beginning of labor with contraction or bleeding, only the cortisone values were found to differ [152]; they were significantly lower in the ruptured membrane group (13.2 ± 3.6 versus 16.3 ± 6.1 μg/liter, $P < 0.05$).

7. 6β, 20β-Dihydroxycortisone

The data available so far are summarized in Table 29. Only in anencephaly are lower values evident. Similar data for normal term deliveries were also described by Drafta et al. [108], and in one case of anencephaly this steroid was not detectable.

Table 29. Concentration of 6β, 20β-dihydroxycortisone in human amniotic fluid in normal and abnormal pregnancies [108, 181]

	6β, 20 β-Dihydroxycortisone (μg/liter)				
	Normal	Diabetes	Rh isoimmunization	Hydramnios	Anencephaly
Case No. 1	0.0	0.0	5.0	0.0	0.0
2	36.0	88.0	5.0	50.0	0.0
3	22.0	58.0	8.0	48.0	0.0
4	20.0	20.0	8.0	33.0	2.0
5	46.0		7.0	17.0	
6	62.0				
Mean	31.0	52.0	7.0	29.0	0.5

8. Other Δ^4-C_{21} Steroids

Only few data are available so far. Corticosterone as the free moiety was found in a pool of normal amniotic fluid in a concentration of 11.3 μg/liter and as sulfate with 48.0 μg/liter [66]. In ten individual measurements, a concentration of the sulfate moiety was found to be 40.0 ± 9.2 μg/liter (mean ± SD) [66]. Similar results were also given in another report [67] with 2.0 μg/liter for the free compound and 38.0 μg/liter for the sulfate. By radioimmunoassay, a range of 2–20 μg/liter was found with no correlation to gestational age [71].

11-Dehydrocorticosterone was also found in the free and sulfate conjugated fraction in a concentration of 1.3 and 18.0 μg/liter, respectively [66]. 11-Deoxycorticosterone was measured as sulfate with 7.0 μg/liter [66]. By radioimmunoassay, no major changes in concentration during the last trimester were found (268). This was also the case for aldosterone [71].

The range was 1–10 μg/liter measuring the 18-oxoglucuronide [71]. More recently, unconjugated aldosterone was measured at 9–20 weeks of gestation with a concentration of 0.14 μg/liter and at 28–40 weeks of gestation with a concentration of 2.1 μg/liter [71a].

No increase could be demonstrated for 11-deoxycortisol when values were compared from 9–20 weeks of gestation (0.6 ng/ml) and from 28–37 weeks of gestation (2.8 ng/ml). Sex differences were not found [70a]. Detailed data for 11-deoxycortisol are shown in Fig. 6 [182].

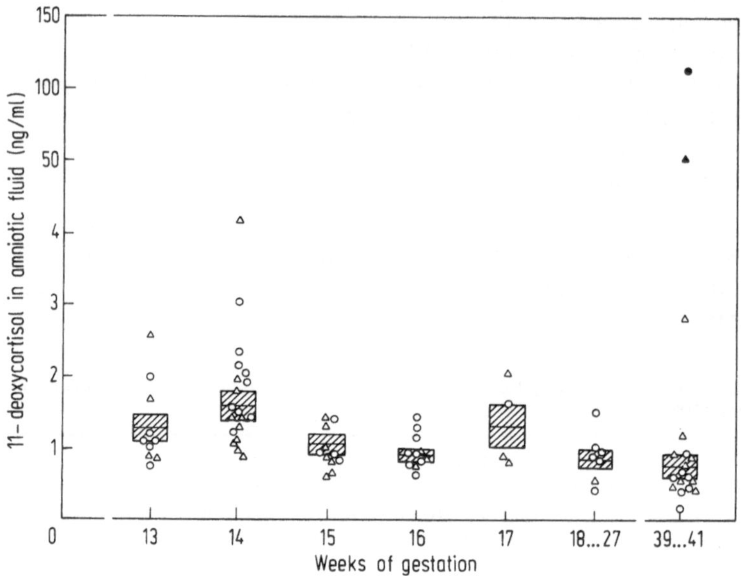

Fig. 6. Amniotic fluid concentrations in normal pregnancies *(open symbols)* and pregnancies carrying fetuses affected with CAH *(closed symbols)*. Males, *triangles*; females, *circles*. The *bars* depict the mean values ± SE (ng/ml). (Schumert et al. 1980 [182])

Significant differences were found between amniotic fluid levels of 11-deoxycortisol at 14 weeks of gestation (1.71 ng/ml) as compared to those at 15 (1.07 ng/ml), 16 (0.94 ng/ml), 18–27 (0.92 ng/ml), and 39–41 (0.83 ng/ml) weeks of gestation ($P < 0.05$). There were no significant differences between samples at 13, 14 and 17 weeks of gestation [182]. No significant differences were found between pregnancies with male fetuses (1.31 ng/ml) and those with female fetuses (1.22 ng/ml). In two pregnancies with fetal congenital adrenal hyperplasia due to 11β-hydroxylase deficiency, the values in amniotic fluid at term were 135 and 64 ng/ml, respectively, as compared to 0.83 ng/ml in 17 normal controls [182]. Similar to 11-deoxycortisol, no change in concentration was found for 21-deoxycortisol (0.21 ng/ml at 9–20 weeks of gestation and 0.23 ng/ml at 28–37 weeks of gestation). Sex differences were not seen [70a]. It was suggested that the measurement of 21-deoxycortisol in human amniotic fluid might help to prenatally detect fetal adrenal 21-hydroxylase deficiency since this compound would be increased in such an abnormality [70a] and would aid other investigative tools, such as 17α-OH-Prog [63, 87, 121, 130, 138] and HLA typing of amniotic cells [70b].

V. Pregnane Steroids

1. Pregnanelone

This steroid has been measured in the glucuronide fraction in a pool of amniotic fluid at term with 43 ± 8 μg/liter [72]. Later in a pool of amniotic fluid at term the concentration was 60 ± 6.0 (SD) μg/liter; in 20 individual samples the concentration was 43.0 ± 4.3 (SEM) μg/liter, while in two pregnancies with an anencephalic fetus similar values (30 and 37 μg/liter) were found [73].

2. Pregnanediol

a) Normal Pregnancies

Data published so far on pregnanediol concentration in amniotic fluid are very limited (Table 30).

Table 30. Method for the determination of pregnanediol in human amniotic fluid

Year of publication	Method	Ref.
1959	Photometry	75
1965	Spectrophotometry	183
1968	GLC	57
1968	GLC	184
1970	GLC	185
1970	GLC	186
1973	Spectrophotometry	187
1975	GLC	72
1979	GLC	73

There appears to be an increase as pregnancy progresses from about 12 μg/liter at 12–17 weeks of gestation [76] to 145 μg/liter near term [57]. In 29 determinations in amniotic fluid from normal pregnancies during the 3rd trimester, a mean concentration of 164.3 ± 22.7 (SEM) μg/liter with a range of 21–447 μg/liter was found [184]. Considerably higher values were measured by authors using spectrophotometric methods [183, 187]. Pennington [183] found in eight cases a mean concentration of 4.26 ± 0.53 (SEM) mg/liter. Woyton et al. [187] determined the values at 35–42 weeks of gestation (Table 31).

Table 31. Human amniotic fluid level of pregnanediol according to Woyton et al. [187]

Weeks of gestation	n	Pregnanediol (mg/liter; mean ± SEM)	P[a]
35–37	11	3.36 ± 0.59	NS
38–41	20	4.37 ± 0.51	<0.001
≧ 42	12	19.25 ± 1.24	

[a] P, Significance

Attention should be directed toward the significantly higher levels at and above 42 weeks of gestation. Whether or not this is connected to the failure of initiation of labor needs to be explored. The relationship of the conjugated and nonconjugated moieties has not been studied systematically. While in early pregnancy 11.9 μg/liter were found in the disulfate fraction [76]; a concentration of 281 µg/liter has been reported in the glucuronide fraction at term [72]. A similar result was recently obtained in a pool of amniotic fluid with 263 ± 35 (SD) µg/liter. In 20 individual samples, the mean concentration was 183 ± 24 (SEM) µg/liter [73].

b) Complicated Pregnancies

In pregnancies complicated by diabetes, hydramnios, anencephaly or severe Rh isoimmunization, the amniotic fluid concentration of pregnanediol did not differ from normal pregnancies [73, 184, 188]. Only in a case of severe Rh isoimmunization with fetal death in utero a very low concentration of 6 µg/liter was found [184]. In uterine fetal growth retardation the values were within the 2.5 and 97.5 percentile limits obtained for a reference group [425].

3. Pregnanetriol

a) Normal Pregnancies

Only few data are available for normal pregnancies (Table 32, Fig. 7). The steroid appears to be present exclusively as sulfate [78].

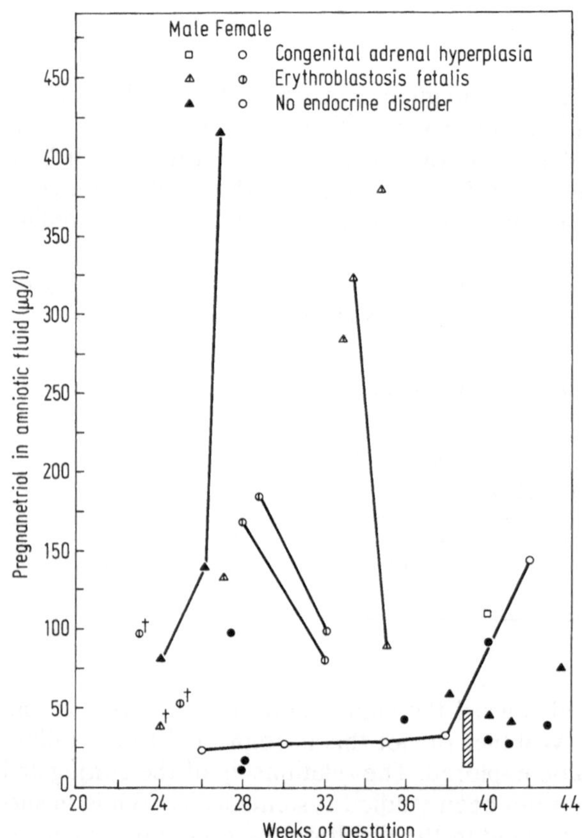

Fig. 7. Variation in amniotic fluid concentration of pregnanetriol during gestation. *Cross-hatched bar* represents the normal range reported by Jeffcoate and associates [77]. The *open square* indicates their finding in a pregnancy resulting in an infant with congenital adrenal hyperplasia. (Merkatz et al. 1969 [189])

Table 32. Concentration of pregnanetriol in normal human amniotic fluid

n	Weeks of gestation	Pregnanetriol (μg/liter)	Ref.
4	39–40	31.2	77
3	40	27.9	78
20	term	60.0	73

b) Complicated Pregnancies

The main purpose of measuring this steroid in amniotic fluid was the prenatal detection of congenital adrenal hyperplasia. Except for the data of Merkatz et al. [189] (for comparison see Fig. 7), the values of normal and affected pregnancies demonstrated an obvious difference (Table 33).

Table 33. Concentration of pregnanetriol in human amniotic fluid with congenital adrenal hyperplasia

Weeks of gestation	n	Pregnanetriol (μg/liter)	Ref.
40	1	106	77
39	1	91	190
40	1	114	191
39	1	206	192
40–2	1	227	
36	1	162	78
40	1	283	

Table 34. Changes of pregnanetriol levels in human amniotic fluid by intra-amniotically injected hydrocortisone on days 278, 280, 283, and 285 [142]

Days of gestation	Pregnanetriol (μg/liter)
277	206
278	277
280	140
283	90
285	22
287 (Delivery)	20

Indeed, by intrauterine treatment with intra-amniotically injected hydrocortisone, a decrease of high pregnanetriol levels could be demonstrated [192] as illustrated in Table 34.

In anencephaly, a low concentration of 11 μg/liter at 39 weeks of gestation was found [77]. In two other cases, the values of 25 and 23 μg/liter were also lower when compared to normal values [73]. As shown in Fig. 7, prior to 36 weeks of gestation fairly high values (> 100 μg/liter) were found [189] in other abnormal conditions and also in normal cases.

4. Other Pregnane Steroids

Besides the data given in a previous chapter on isolation and identification of steroids in amniotic fluid, further quantitative measurements of THF and THE in normal pregnancies were done by radioimmunoassay, indicating a rise after 30 weeks of gestation [71].

A good correlation between THF and THE values in amniotic fluid was found (r = 0.682). In cases of RDS of the fetus, the values were low [71]. Further data have been obtained by a recent study [79] as listed in Table 35.

Table 35. THF, THE, and THS in human amniotic fluid (μg/liter; mean ± SD) [419]

Weeks of gestation	n	THF	THE	THS
14 –26.5	100	5.8 ± 3.3	6.1 ± 3.6	7.1 ± 4.2
26.5–41	25	17.0 ± 13.1	27.8 ± 15.1	22.6 ± 10.7

In two pregnancies with fetuses affected by 11β-hydroxylase deficiency evaluated at 18 and 40 weeks of gestation, respectively, the following data were obtained: THF: 9.8 and 24.0 μg/liter; THE: 10.5 and 26.0 μg/liter; THS: 89 and 189 μg/liter. Thus, only THS was significantly higher in amniotic fluid when compared to normal controls. A significantly elevated $\frac{\text{THS}}{\text{THF} + \text{THE}}$ ratio was also found in pregnancies with affected fetuses [79].

The data suggest that the diagnosis of 11β-hydroxylase deficiency may be established more precisely during pregnancy than within the first 2 weeks of gestation if there are no clinical features of the disease in the newborn [79].

Some data are available on other pregnane steroids measured at term (Table 36).

Table 36. Pregnane glucuronides in human amniotic fluid at term (μg/liter) [73]

	5β-pregnan-20-one-3α,6α-diol	5α-pregnan-20-one-3α,16α-diol
At term	48 ± 6[a]	161 ± 20[a]
Anencephaly		
Case No. 1	54	92
Case No. 2	36	60

[a] Mean ± SEM

VI. 17-Hydroxycorticosteroids

a) Normal Pregnancies

A first report on 17-hydroxycorticoids in human amniotic fluid at term was given by Pennington [183]. In 26 samples, he found a mean concentration of 780 ± 100 (SEM) μg/liter with a range of 0.0–2,000 μg/liter. In a more detailed investigation, Wade and Abramovich [193] found generally lower concentrations. Details are given in Table 37.

Table 37. Concentrations of 17-hydroxycorticosteroids in human amniotic fluid

Weeks of gestation	Fetal sex	n	17-Hydroxycortico-steroids (μg/liter)	Ref.
11–19	Male	8	58.3	194
	Female	8	48.2	
26–36	Male/Female	10	145.3	194
At term	Male	10	255.5	193
	Female	10	224.5	

In early pregnancy (11–19 weeks of gestation), lower concentrations were found [194]. In 16 cases, a normal level of 53.2 ± 15.7 (SEM) μg/liter was measured. Similar to the values at term (Table 36), the concentration was slightly higher for males than for females (58.3 ± 13.8 versus 48.2 ± 16.8 μg/liter). Between 26–36 weeks of gestation, there was an increase to an average concentration of 145.3 μg/liter [194], but some of these pregnancies were abnormal.

b) Complicated Pregnancies

In anencephaly [193], a low level of 17-hydroxycorticosteroids in amniotic fluid has been found (57 versus 240 μg/liter). Taking average amniotic fluid volumes for normal and anencephalic pregnancies as described by Gadd [195], differences in total concentration were not found, but such an approach would only be valid if the actual amniotic fluid volume for each pregnancy is taken into account. In amniotic fluid from an adrenalectomized patient at 38 weeks of gestation, a low concentration was also found (174.2 μg/liter).

VII. 11-Hydroxycorticosteroids

To date, two reports give data on 11-hydroxycorticosteroids determined in amniotic fluid [196, 197]. In contrast to the higher androgen levels found in human amniotic fluid with a male fetus (see corresponding chapter), this steroid was found to be present in a significantly ($P < 0.01$) lower concentration in pregnancies with male fetuses [196] (Table 38).

Throughout normal pregnancy, a significant rise of 11-hydroxycorticosteroids was reported by Mukherjee et al. [197] as demonstrated in Fig. 8.

However, when amniotic fluid from both normal and abnormal pregnancies were analyzed according to the weeks of gestation, the correlation was less between 38–45 weeks of gestation (see Fig. 8).

Prior to onset of spontaneous labor, a rise of the corticosteroid level in amniotic fluid was found that was not obvious when delivery was done by

Table 38. Concentration of unconjugated 11-hydroxycorticosteroids in human amniotic fluid [196]

	Unconjugated 11-hydroxycorticosteroids (μg/liter)	
	Male fetus	Female fetus
Case No. 1	60	87
2	50	40
3	43	70
4	35	70
5	34	113
6	40	33
7	39	60
8	40	43
9	40	56
10	26	80
11	36	50
12	30	105
13	53	46
14	20	43
15	53	129
16	56	–
17	36	–
Mean	43.1	65.0
SD	±10.6	±29.0
P[a] <0.01		

[a] P, Significance of sex difference

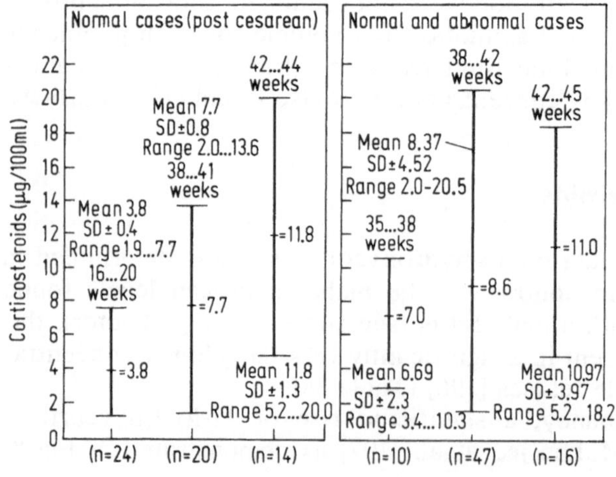

Fig. 8. Corticosteroid levels in amniotic fluid in different periods of gestation in normal and abnormal cases. The mean, range, and standard deviations are given for each group in different periods of gestation. (Mukherjee et al. 1977 [197])

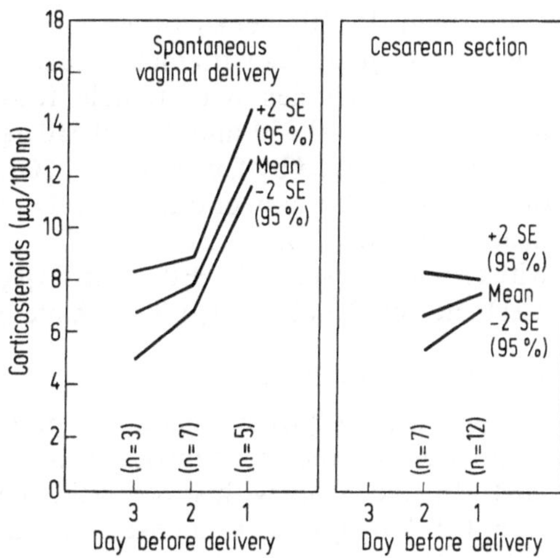

Fig. 9. Amniotic fluid corticosteroid levels prior to the date of delivery in spontaneous vaginal delivery and cesarean section. (Mukherjee et al. 1977 [197])

cesarean section as shown in Fig. 9. Furthermore, a significant correlation ($P < 0.0001$) between birth weights of babies born spontaneously and the corticosteroid level in amniotic fluid was noted [197]. Such a correlation was not present when cesarean section was performed [197].

VIII. Δ^5-C_{19} Steroids

1. Dehydroepiandrosterone (D)

a) Normal Pregnancies

Similar results were obtained for total D in pooled and single samples of normal third trimester pregnancies [57, 184]. In one 4 liter pool, the concentration was 8.3 µg/liter [57] and in 14 samples the concentration was 7.0 ± 1.9 (SEM) µg/liter with a range of 0.5–17.3 µg/liter [184]. Gandy [89] differentiated between D and DS and found concentrations of 0.5 (range 0.4–0.6) and 5.4 µg/liter (range 4.8 ± 5.9), respectively. DS was recently measured in a 1 liter pool with 10 µg/liter [82].

A detailed study [198] for free D throughout gestation according to male and female fetuses has been done with RIA. The data are listed in Table 39, indicating no major change throughout gestation with male and female fetuses.

Table 39. Free dehydroepiandrosterone in human amniotic fluid [198]

Weeks of gestation	Free dehydroepiandrosterone (µg/liter; mean ± SEM)	
	Male fetus	Female fetus
8–12	0.315 ± 0.071	0.310 ± 0.050
12–15	0.322 ± 0.058	0.358 ± 0.037
16–20	$0.416 + 0.063$	0.329 ± 0.085
32–40	0.329 ± 0.085	–

Between 15–20 weeks of gestation, this was also confirmed by others [199]. In pregnancies with male fetuses, the level of D was 0.230 ± 0.02 (SEM) and for pregnancies with female fetuses 0.210 ± 0.02 (SEM) μg/liter with a range of 0.06–0.350 and 0.08–0.510 μg/liter, respectively [199]. Similar data were also reported by Dvorák et al. [200]. In pregnancies between 14–22 weeks of gestation, the concentration of D in 26 samples from pregnancies with a male fetus was 0.184 ± 0.096 (SD) and in 24 samples from pregnancies with female fetuses 0.177 ± 0.012 (SD) μg/liter. Higher values for D (1.5–15.0 μg/liter) and for DS (20–200 μg/liter) have been reported by others [177, 201].

b) Complicated Pregnancies

In diabetes, polyhydramnios, or pregnancies severely affected by Rh incompatibility, the concentration of total D was similar to normal cases [184]. In five cases with severe Rh isoimmunization, the concentration ranged from 0.5–7.6 μg/liter. In a case of intrauterine fetal death due to Rh incompatibility, D could not be detected [184]. Saez and Bertrand [88] described in two pools of amniotic fluid from male fetuses between 33–35 and 37–38 weeks of gestation as well as in two pools of female fetuses between 32–33 and 36–38 weeks of gestation concentrations below 10 μg/liter. All pregnancies were affected by Rh incompatibility.

Using RIA, DS was determined in amniotic fluid in a case with placental sulfatase deficiency [178]. A concentration of 450 μg/liter was measured, and in three control cases a mean of 47.3 μg/liter with a range of 22–60 μg/liter was found indicating that the steroid levels in amniotic fluid reflect the inability of the placenta to metabolize fetal DS, leading to accumulation in the fetal circulation and increased passage into the amniotic fluid. In another case with placental sulfatase deficiency, D was found in a concentration of 63 μg/liter [202]; in a further report [177], DS was found to be extremely high (2,400 μg/liter) when compared to the normal range of 20–200 μg/liter. The D level with 2.0 μg/liter was not different from a normal range of 1.5–15.0 μg/liter [201]. In a case with fetal adrenal hypoplasia, D was below 0.2 μg/liter and DS below 5 μg/liter [201].

2. Androst-5-ene-3β,17α-diol and Androst-5-ene-3β,17β-diol

Both steroids increase in the disulfate fraction from early and midtrimester toward term from 6.3 and 2.6 μg/liter to 224 and 42 μg/liter, respectively [59, 76]. The latter steroid was measured in nine normal pregnancies in a concentration of 56 μg/liter with a range of 0–80 μg/liter [203]. In three cases of anencephaly, the concentration ranged from 3–11 μg/liter and 2–8 μg/liter, respectively [103], indicating that the fetal adrenal determines mainly the amniotic fluid content of both steroids. In gestosis, androst-5-ene,3β,17β-diol was found with a mean concentration of 103 μg/liter (range 0–220 μg/liter) [203].

In a recent study [204], Δ^5-androstene-3β,17α-diol was measured from the 24th week of gestation until term in normal pregnancies, demonstrating an increasing level of the steroid ranging from 20 to 100 μg/liter.

In complicated pregnancies, the concentrations of this steroid were lower than in normal cases and directly related to the severity of the pathologic

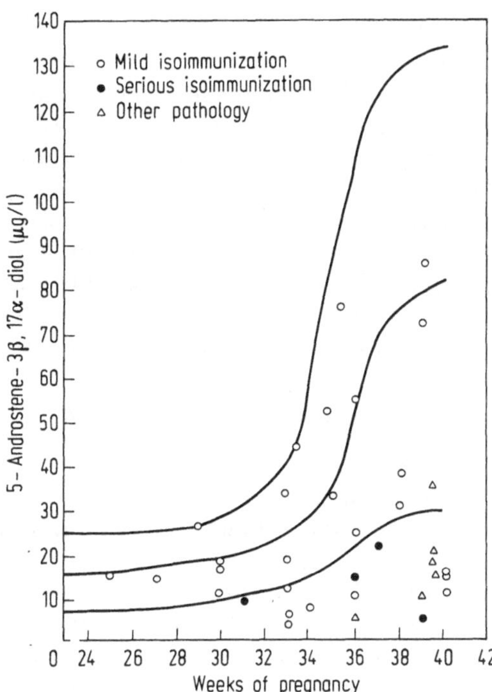

Fig. 10. 5-Androstene-3β,17α-diol levels in amniotic fluid in some cases of pathologic pregnancy. (Mancuso et al. 1980 [204])

situation [204]. This was particularly helpful in cases with severe Rh isoimmunization where repeated amniocenteses and intrauterine blood transfusions made bilirubin assay unusable for prognostic purposes (see Fig. 10).

3. **16α-Hydroxydehydroepiandrosterone** (16-OH-D)

a) Normal Pregnancies

In early and midtrimester pregnancies, a concentration of 8.2 μg/liter was found in the disulfate fraction [76]. At term, total 16-OH-D was quantitated from amniotic fluid pools with a concentration of 797 [57] and 1,020 μg/liter [81]. Similar levels were detected in individual samples with a mean concentration of 599.6 ± 104 (SEM) μg/liter (n = 18) and a range of 75–1,528 μg/liter [184] and in nine cases with a mean concentration of 119 μg/liter and a range of 55–200 μg/liter [203]. In 20 samples at term, 16-OH-DS was present in a concentration of 165 ± 41 (SEM) μg/liter. Menini and Bellarti [205] measured this steroid from 32 weeks of gestation until the 43rd week of gestation and noted a considerable increase toward term; 32–36 weeks of gestation, a mean concentration of 246 μg/liter (n = 6) and a range of 80–602 μg/liter was present. Between 40–43 weeks of gestation, the range was 75–1,230 μg/liter, resulting in a mean value of 477 μg/liter (n = 11).
In another study, lower values were measured although 16-OH-D and 16-keto-A were determined together [108], but these data were not corrected for losses. There was a mean concentration of 217.9 ± 42.4 (SEM) μg/liter (n = 11) with a range of 64–493 μg/liter [108]. Recently 16-OH-D was measured in pooled amniotic fluid at 160 μg/liter [82].

b) Complicated Pregnancies

In severe Rh isoimmunization, this steroid could not be detected in amniotic fluid [184]. Similar results were obtained by Menini and Bellarti [205] who could find little or none of this estriol precursor in amniotic fluid. In diabetes and hydramnios, values were measured at 145 and 80 μg/liter, respectively [184]. In placenta sulfatase deficiency, a mean sulfate concentration of 450 μg/liter with a range of 30–7,750 μg/liter was reported [82]. In gestosis, a mean concentration of 345 μg/liter with a range of 233–481 μg/liter was found [203]. However, in anencephaly this steroid was undetectable [73, 184]. Three of 12 pregnancies with intruaterine fetal growth retardation demonstrated amniotic fluid values below the 2.5 percentile [445].

4. **16-Ketoandrostenediol** (16-keto-A)

a) Normal Pregnancies

In pools of normal amniotic fluid at term, concentrations between 575 [57] and 1,100 μg/liter [81] were reported, with an increase from the first and second trimester of pregnancy of 15 μg/liter found in the disulfate fraction [76]. At term, only 6 μg/liter were measured in the disulfate fraction [59], while the sulfate fraction was quantitated in pooled amniotic fluid at 40 μg/liter [82], and the sulfate and sulfoglucuronide fractions revealed 46 μg/liter [73]. In single samples throughout the third trimester of normal pregnancy ($n = 13$), the concentration ranged between 20 and 471 μg/liter with a mean of 210.9 ± 35.0 (SEM) μg/liter [184]. Others found between the 33rd and 36th weeks of gestation concentrations between 86 and 280 μg/liter and between the 41st and 43rd weeks of gestation, a range of 90–860 μg/liter [205]. At term, the sulfate and sulfoglucuronide fractions in 20 samples contained a concentration of 53 ± 5.3 (SEM) μg/liter [73].

b) Complicated Pregnancies

Only limited data are available in complicated pregnancies. In severe Rh isoimmunization, this steroid was not found in amniotic fluid by two independent studies [184, 205]. It was measured in one case with diabetes mellitus and in a case of polyhydramnios at 34 μg/liter [184]. In placental sulfatase deficiency, a concentration of 180 μg/liter was found as sulfate [82].

5. **16,18-Dihydroxydehydroepiandrosterone**

Only one report contains data on this steroid as sulfate moiety in human amniotic fluid [82]. In normal pooled amniotic fluid, 40 μg/liter was found and in three cases with placental sulfatase deficiency a range of 10–3,520 μg/liter (mean 190 μg/liter) was measured [82].

6. **Androstenetriol** (A-triol)

a) Normal Pregnancies

Besides the measurements in pooled amniotic fluid at term with 48 [57] and 30 μg/liter [82] as sulfate, only one study reports on the determination in single samples where a concentration of 100.0 ± 18.6 (SEM) μg/liter with a range of 50–142 μg/liter was found [108].

b) Complicated Pregnancies

In only one pregnancy with anencephaly was the attempt made to measure A-triol, but it was not detected [108]. In three cases with placental sulfatase deficiency, the sulfate fraction of A-triol contained 120 μg/liter with a range of 10–5,520 μg/liter [82].

IX. Δ^4-C_{19} Steroids

1. Androstenedione

Interest has mainly been focused on the determination of this steroid in early pregnancy to delineate sex differences. The data are summarized in Table 40.

Table 40. Androstenedione concentration in human amniotic fluid

Weeks of gestation	Fetal sex	n	Androstenedione (μg/liter; mean ± SEM)	P[a]	Ref.
14–20	Male	48	1.04 ± 0.05	<0.001	83, 199
	Female	72	0.66 ± 0.03		
14–18	Male	66	0.658 ± 0.03	<0.001	85
	Female	33	0.360 ± 0.02		
14–20	Male	76	0.348 ± 0.032	<0.05	87
	Female	76	0.156 ± 0.029		
26–40	Male	25	0.187 ± 0.027	<0.05	87
	Female		0.331 ± 0.038		
12–20	–	–	0.871	–	84
–	–	–	0.12 0.1–0.14[b]	–	89
–	–	–	0.7–3.5[b]	–	201

[a] P, Significance of sex differences
[b] Range

Besides the evaluation of a sex difference of androstenedione in amniotic fluid, further clinical studies regarding the compound had been done in nine normal pregnancies and in nine pregnancies with gestosis [203] revealing a concentration of 9.0 μg/liter (range 0–15) and 17.0 μg/liter (range 0–30), respectively. These values are considerably higher than those reported by others [87], which is most likely due to lack of specificity of the method. In a case with congenital adrenal hyperplasia, three consecutive measurements yielded only one value above the normal range [87]. In a pregnancy with congenital fetal adrenal hypoplasia the value for A in amniotic fluid was 1.5 μg/liter compared to the normal range of 0.7–8.5 μg/liter [206]. In a case with hydatidiform degeneration of the placenta, no differences from normal were seen [87].

2. Testosterone

a) Normal Pregnancies

Measurements of testosterone in amniotic fluid have been carried out fairly extensively, primarily focusing on sex differences in concentration. Such differences were first noted in pools of amniotic fluid [88]. This was found for the free and sulfate fraction of testosterone [88] as listed in Table 41.

Table 41. Concentration of testosterone and testosterone sulfate in human amniotic fluid [88]

	Weeks of gestation	Testosterone (pg/100 ml)	Testosterone sulfate (pg/100 ml)
I Pool male fetus	37–38	67	178
II Pool male fetus	33–35	55	198
I Pool female fetus	32–33	35	141
II Pool female fetus	36–38	25	67

Later on, numerous data were published using a variety of methods at different times throughout gestation. The data are compiled in Table 42. The type of testosterone fraction measured is indicated. While Stahl et al. [90] found significant differences at term for the free and glucoronide fractions, the result of the investigation of Younglai [208] was that total 17β-hydroxy androgens at term cannot be used as an indicator of the sex of the fetus.

Besides the sex differences, there is also a change in testosterone concentration in amniotic fluid during the course of pregnancy. Judd et al. [93] measured the highest values for testosterone in amniotic fluid in pregnancies with male fetuses in the 17th and 18th weeks of gestation. No elevation of the testosterone levels was noted in pregnancies with female fetuses. A decrease toward term is obvious in pregnancies with male fetuses [87, 92, 96, 99, 100]. Most of the published data demonstrate significant differences of testosterone levels in amniotic fluid in human gestation with male and female fetuses (see Table 41). These differences seem to be missing prior to the 12th week of gestation and become less pronounced toward term [87, 92, 98, 99, 102]. This is in full agreement with data on testosterone in cord blood [207, 212, 213]. However, because of overlap, definite sex determination from levels of testosterone in amniotic fluid cannot be made in all cases. The possible prediction of fetal sex from testosterone levels in amniotic fluid range from 45% [210] to 100%, particularly when these measurements are done at midgestation [86, 92, 93].

Variations in values are dependent on sensitivity and specificity of the assays using different antisera and chromatographic steps and in part on the hydrolysis step used to measure total immunoreactive 17β-hydroxyandrogens [92].

Table 42. Testosterone in human amniotic fluid

Weeks of gestation	Fetal sex	n	Testosterone (pg/ml)		P[0]	Method	Ref.
			Mean ± SEM, SD	Range			
Term	Male	17	4320 ± 1200 SD[b]	2200–7200	<0.001	Protein binding	90
	Female	15	2310 ± 1200 SD[b]	850–5450			
12–20	Male	60	206 ± 7,6 SEM[c]	710– 383	<0.025	RIA	208
	Female	39	173 ± 10,0 SEM[c]	80– 375			
12–20	Male	7	286 ± 198 SD[a]	–	NS	Protein binding	209
	Female	5	224 ± 102 SD[a]	–			
10–12	Male	24	1334 ± 366 SD[b]	860–2030	<0.001	RIA	91
13–28			2130 ± 357 SD[b]	1820–2520			
29–40			2282 ± 989 SD[b]	1130–4020	<0.002		
10–12	Female	17	463 ± 328 SD[b]	160–1080	<0.05		
13–28			780 ± 220 SD[b]	520–1000	<0.05		
29–40			1225 ± 635 SD[b]	730–2360			
16–20	Male	38	176 ± 8 SEM[d]	105– 329	<0.05	RIA	92
	Female	19	60 ± 5 SEM[d]	24– 90			
Term	Male	37	123 ± 12 SD[d]	94– 290	<0.05		
	Female	38	63 ± 4 SD[d]	33– 96			
15–25	Male	58	223 ± 10 SD[a]	104– 424	<0.001	RIA	93
	Female	77	40 ± 2 SEM[a]	18– 82			

[a] Free
[b] Free and glucuronide fraction
[c] Free, conjugated, and protein-bound testosterone
[d] Glucuronide
[0] P, Significance of sex differences

Continued next page

Table 42 (continued)

Weeks of gestation	Fetal sex	n	Testosterone (pg/ml)		P^0	Method	Ref.
			Mean ± SEM, SD	Range			
14–20	Male	73	202[a]	–	<0.001	RIA	94
	Female	49	41[a]	–			
14–20	Male	24	267[d]	–	<0.05		
	Female	18	123[e]	–			
14–20	Male	13	480[e]	–	NS		
	Female	8	425[e]	–			
16–26	Male	11	1038 ± 345 SD[d]	710–1830	<0.001	RIA	95
	Female	9	435 ± 140 SD[d]				
16–26	Male	8	292 ± 143 SD[a]	130– 560	<0.01		
	Female	9	84 ± 23 SD[a]	60– 140			
12–15	Male	21	501 ± 185 SD[a]	224–1004	<0.0005	RIA	96
	Female	20	281 ± 74 SD[a]	93– 304			
16–20	Male	55	427 ± 128 SD[a]	240– 721	<0.0005		
	Female	41	201 ± 53 SD[a]	100– 300			
21–30	Male	16	374 ± 129 SD[a]	204– 613	<0.0025		
	Female	8	183 ± 44 SD[a]	119– 464			
31–42	Male	21	281 ± 74 SD[a]	192– 464	<0.005		
	Female	10	186 ± 36 SD[a]	161– 248			
14–20	Male	48	222 ± 11 SEM[a]	–	<0.001	RIA	83
	Female	72	39 ± 2 SEM[a]	–			199
14–22	Male	66	277 ± 16 SEM[a]	–	<0.001		85
	Female	33	41 ± 3 SEM[a]	–			86
10–20	Male	31	168 ± 95 SD[a]	20– 390	<0.001	RIA	97
	Female	23	44 ± 26 SD[a]	20– 90			
Up to 25	Male	69	165 ± 15 SEM[a]	30– 592	<0.001	RIA	98

9–12	Male	6	50[a]	2– 726	NS	RIA	99
	Female	2	27[a]	13– 46			
12–16	Male	16	250[a]	70– 724	<0.0001		
	Female	17	26[a]	13– 100			
16–19	Male	10	193[a]	84– 290	<0.0001		
	Female	14	29[a]	10– 90			
34–40	Male	11	80[a]	20– 160	<0.02		
	Female	10	34[a]	22– 102			
Up to 20	Male	8	199 ± 82 SD[a]	93– 320	<0.005	RIA	100
	Female	6	75 ± 32 SD[a]	39– 123			
21–30	Male	13	222 ± 97 SD[a]	134– 395	<0.001		
	Female	10	68 ± 23 SD[a]	36– 103			
31–40	Male	10	149 ± 48 SD[a]	99– 262	<0.001		
	Female	10	60 ± 21 SD[a]	40– 97			
16–19	Male		276[a]	155– 413	<0.001	RIA	101
	Female		96[a]	57– 151			
15–19	Male	60	170.6 ± 60.2 SD[a]		<0.001	RIA	102
	Female	51	41.9 ± 20.3 SD[a]				
14–20	Male	–	188 ± 1.4 SEM[a]	86– 477	<0.001	RIA	87
	Female	–	22 ± 2 SEM[a]	6– 64			
26–40	Male	–	107 ± 15 SEM[a]	68– 172	<0.001	RIA	87
	Female	–	56 ± 9 SEM[a]	21– 132			
16–20	Male	402	363 ± 108 SD[a]	–	–	RIA	210
	Female	410	180 ± 41 SD[a]	–			
15–19	Male	62	162 ± 7 SD[a]	–	<0.0005	RIA	24
	Female	39	60 ± 2 SD[a]	–			
14–22	Male	26	249 ± 109 SD[a]	–	<0.001	RIA	200
	Female	24	70 ± 38 SD[a]	–			

[e] Sulfate

The importance of the type of testosterone assay approach was recently demonstrated [102]. Quantitation of T in amniotic fluid without chromatographic separation prior to RIA resulted in a considerable overlap of the values for pregnancies with male and female fetuses. The data are listed in Table 43, which demonstrates that there are significant differences between the T values with and without chromatograph for both sexes ($P < 0.001$).

Table 43. Determination of testosterone in human amniotic fluid with and without chromatography [102]

Fetal sex	n	Testosterone (pg/ml; mean ± SD)		$\frac{T}{iT} \times 100$ (%)
		With chromatography (T)	Without chromatography (iT)	
Male	60	170.6 ± 60.2	565.8 ± 129.0	30.2 ± 8.3
Female	51	41.9 ± 20.3	298.2 ± 77.1	14.1 ± 6.5

b) Complicated Pregnancies

Except for a group of patients with Rh incompatibility [209], no specific studies have been carried out in complicated pregnancies. Data on some single cases are variable. In two cases with congenital adrenal hyperplasia, testosterone in amniotic fluid did not allow differentiation from normal [87, 209]. In a pregnancy with a male fetus homogenous for Tay-Sachs disease and a female fetus with Gaucher disease, the testosterone level was within the range of normal for the appropriate sex and age of gestation [93]. However, a male fetus with a XXY chromosome constitution had a value for testosterone in amniotic fluid in the female range, indicating abnormal fetal testicular development [96].

X. Androstane Steroids

1. Dihydrotestosterone (DHT)

So far DHT has only been measurable in amniotic fluid specimens with male fetuses [87]. Between 14–20 weeks of gestation, the levels ranged between 0.008 and 0.067 ng/ml (mean 0.024 ± 0.003 ng/ml) and for 26–40 weeks of gestation between 0.011 and 0.064 ng/ml (mean 0.026 ± 0.006 ng/ml). DHT was also detected in a case with congenital adrenal hyperplasia and in a case with hydatidiform degeneration of the placenta [87].

XI. 17-Ketosteroids

a) Normal Pregnancies

Spectrophotometric estimations of 17-ketosteroids were first reported in 1965 [183]. High values were found by Pennington (range 1.0–4.5 mg/liter, mean 2.7 mg/liter) most likely due to lack of sufficient purification [183].

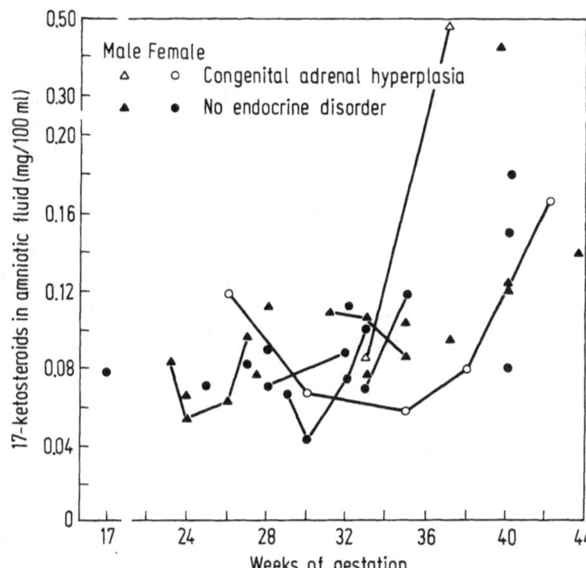

Fig. 11. Variation in amniotic fluid concentration of 17-ketosteroids during gestation. (Merkatz et al. 1969 [189])

Using alumina column chromatography and micro-Zimmermann reaction, concentrations between 25 and 52 μg/liter (mean 38 μg/liter) were found in normal pregnancies between 39 and 40 weeks of gestation [77]. A detailed study by Wade and Abramovich in 1967 [193] of 20 amniotic fluid samples gave an average value of 119.8 μg/liter.

A sex difference was not found. This was also confirmed by the data of Merkatz et al. [189]. These values are higher and show an increase toward term (Fig. 11). In early pregnancy (11–19 weeks of gestation), lower values were described [194].

Again no sex differences were present as shown in Table 44. Between 26 and 36 weeks of gestation, the average value rose to 74.4 μg/liter. This group consisted in part of complicated pregnancies [194].

Table 44. 17-Ketosteroids in human amniotic fluid [193, 194]

Weeks of gestation	17-Ketosteroids (μg/liter; mean ± SEM)						Ref.
	Male fetus	n	Female fetus	n	Total	n	
11–19	44.0 ± 4.3	11	38.7 ± 5.1	8	41.8 ± 3.2	19	194
At term	116.4	10	121.9	10	119.8	20	193

b) Complicated Pregnancies

The clinical usefulness of measurements of 17-ketosteroid in amniotic fluid was pointed out by Jeffcoate et al. [77], indicating elevated levels in pregnancies with fetuses affected by congenital adrenal hyperplasia (104 versus 38 μg/liter in normals) and low levels in anencephaly (16 μg/liter). This was confirmed by others [193]. The range of values was 28–38 μg/liter. These authors pointed out, however, that taking the total volume of amniotic fluid into account, the total amount of 17-ketosteroids is similar to normal cases [193]. Whether such an approach is valid remains to be determined since in other instances normal concentrations have been found in spite of hydramnios [184] and low levels persisted in spite of taking the amniotic fluid volume into account [214]. In one case, the concentration of 17-ketosteroids in amniotic fluid in early and late gestation did not distinguish the affected from the unaffected fetuses [189]. In an adrenalectomized patient at 38 weeks gestation, the 17-ketosteroid concentration in amniotic fluid was not different from normal pregnancy [215], indicating that the 17-ketosteroid content of amniotic fluid is mainly determined by the fetus.

XII. C_{18} Steroids

1. Estrone

a) Normal Pregnancies

No major change of this steroid in human amniotic fluid appears to occur during pregnancy. Twenty years ago, values of 2.5–4.4 μg/liter from 15 weeks of gestation to term had already been reported [104, 105]. The value of free versus total estrone in amniotic fluid was 0.8 versus 2.5 μg/liter up to the 25th week of gestation and at term 0.9 versus 4.4 μg/liter [105]. Others have found values at term of 5.6 versus 8.0 μg/liter in seven pooled amniotic fluid samples [109]. Further studies reported a concentration of 2.3–4.0 μg/liter at term [81] and 9.0 μg/liter for six samples between the 38th and 42nd weeks of gestation [107]; in 12 samples, 5.0 μg/liter were described [216]. In nine cases, a mean concentration of E_1 of 7.0 μg/liter with a range of 3–13 μg/liter was determined [203].

Total estrone measured by the method of Brown near term resulted in a concentration of 48.5 ± 4.6 (SEM) μg/liter [108]. Using specific RIA, free estrone in amniotic fluid has been measured in early and late pregnancy and according to the sex of the fetus.

Mennuti et al. [86] described free estrone in amniotic fluid from 14–22 weeks of gestation to be 0.256 ± 0.018 μg/liter (mean ± SEM) in males and 0.303 ± 0.030 μg/liter in females. Others [83, 199] have found levels to be significantly higher in pregnancies with male fetuses (0.353 ± 0.033 versus 0.331 ± 0.028 μg/liter). The difference was not significant.

b) Complicated Pregnancies

In anencephaly, the concentration of estrone in amniotic fluid at 0.9 μg/liter was found to be ten times lower than in normal pregnancy [107]. In diabetes mellitus [106], fairly high values were reported for free estrone [19.9 ± 4.3 (SD) μg/liter, n = 12], but a normal group was not studied with the same method. Our own data are summarized in Table 45. There are on the average lower values in Rh incompatibility. In edema, diabetes, and premature labor, no differences were found (Table 46). Betamethasone or dexamethasone treatment in groups of pregnant women at risk did not reveal significant changes [131, 135] as shown in Table 47.

Table 45. Unconjugated estrone in normal human amniotic fluid [129]

Weeks of gestation	n	Unconjugated estrone (μg/liter; mean ± SEM)
9–16	10	1.16 ± 0.06
38	2	3.00 ± 1.20
39	3	3.62 ± 0.86
40	9	2.66 ± 0.24
41	3	2.93 ± 0.96
42	6	2.05 ± 0.24

Table 46. Estrone in human amniotic fluid in various clinical disorders [129]

Weeks of gestation	Estrone (μg/liter; mean ± SEM)							
	Edema	n	Rh incompatibility	n	Diabetes	n	Premature labor	n
28–31	1.30 ± 0.10	7	1.28 ± 0.10	10	–	–	1.25 ± 0.05	3
32–34	1.62 ± 0.29	7	1.19 ± 0.19	13	–	–	1.15 ± 0.12	4
35–37	1.28 ± 0.23	11	1.02 ± 0.09	13	1.40 ± 0.38	2	1.14 ± 0.20	14
38	1.68 ± 0.27	11	1.08 ± 0.17	4	1.24 ± 0.36	2	1.34 ± 0.33	3
39	2.42 ± 0.78	5	1.06 ± 0.11	2	1.75	1	–	–
40	1.93 ± 0.23	11	–	–	–	–	2.21 ± 0.47	4
41	2.65 ± 0.54	8	–	–	1.78 ± 0.32	2	1.71 ± 0.57	2
42	2.42 ± 0.99	4	–	–	–	–	–	–

Table 47. Estrone and estradiol in human amniotic fluid (μg/liter) before and after betamethasone and dexamethasone treatment [131, 135]

	n	Amniocentesis I		Amniocentesis II		Ref.
		E_1	E_2	E_1	E_2	
Betamethasone group[a]	10	0.52 ± 0.10	0.51 ± 0.08	0.33 ± 0.05	0.52 ± 0.17	131
Control group[a]	5	0.48 ± 0.13	0.34 ± 0.10	0.52 ± 0.12	0.36 ± 0.07	
Dexamethasone group[b]	10	0.44 ± 0.15	0.46 ± 0.26	0.45 ± 0.13	0.47 ± 0.36	135

[a] Values = Mean ± SEM
[b] Values = Mean ± SD

2. Estradiol-17β

a) Normal Pregnancies

Similar to estrone, the change of estradiol in amniotic fluid during the course of pregnancy is small from 1.2 to 3.1 μg/liter [105]. In early studies, free and conjugated estradiol could not even be quantitated [104]. Later on, values at term were reported: 9.0 [107], 2.0 [216], 1.4 [109], and 0.8–1.9 μg/liter [81]. Low levels for free E_2 determined by RIA in human amniotic fluid were found by a number of investigators [83, 86, 87, 199]. The data are summarized in Table 48.

Table 48. Free estradiol in normal human amniotic fluid

Weeks of gestation	Estradiol (μg/liter)				Ref.
	Male	n	Female	n	
14–22	0.085	66	0.102	33	86
14–20	0.036	–	0.048	–	87
26–40	0.043	–	0.067	–	
14–20	0.064	48	0.096	72	83, 199

The portion of free versus total estradiol appears to be high with 2.1 versus 3.1 μg/liter [105]. Others were able to find trace amounts of free estradiol and 1.4 μg/liter as the conjugated moiety [141]. Higher values near term were reported by Drafta et al. [108] who measured total estradiol by the method of Brown. In 24 samples, the mean concentration was 51.5 ± 6.8 (SEM) μg/liter. In early and late pregnancy, free estradiol was quantitated by RIA as shown in Table 49.

An extensive study by Warne et al. [198] on the relationship of E_2 levels in amniotic fluid to fetal sex and age is shown in Table 50.

Table 49. Free estradiol in normal human amniotic fluid [129]

Weeks of gestation	n	Free estradiol (μg/liter; mean ± SEM)
9–16	10	0.43 ± 0.05
38	2	1.63 ± 1.07
39	3	1.60 ± 0.38
40	9	1.34 ± 0.19
41	3	1.06 ± 0.04
42	6	0.94 ± 0.10

Table 50. Free estradiol in human amniotic fluid [198]

Weeks of gestation	Free estradiol (μg/liter)	
	Male fetus	Female fetus
8–11	0.85	0.56
12–15	0.35	0.40
16–20	0.32	0.32
32–40	1.72	1.15

b) Complicated Pregnancies

Similar to estrone, low values were also found in anencephaly for estradiol: 2.0 versus 9.0 μg/liter in normal pregnancy [107]. Relatively high values have been measured in diabetes mellitus [14.9 ± 3.7 (SD) μg/liter, $n = 12$], but no control group has been studied [106]. Lower values were found in Rh incompatibility. In diabetes and premature labor, no differences were found. In three cases with placental insufficiency, the E_2 values were similar to the normal group when compared to the values determined in the same assay system [87]. In a pregnancy with a cephalothoracopagus, the E_2 concentration in amniotic fluid was found to be 1.3 μg/liter at 28 weeks of gestation [179]. Under betamethasone or dexamethasone treatment, no changes have been noted in pregnant patients at risk. A summary of our own data is compiled in Table 51.

Table 51. Estradiol in human amniotic fluid in various clinical disorders [129]

Weeks of gestation	Estradiol (μg/liter; mean ± SEM)							
	Edema	n	Rh incompatibility	n	Diabetes	n	Premature labor	n
28–31	0.31 ± 0.05	7	0.27 ± 0.03	10	–	–	0.37 ± 0.008	3
32–34	0.30 ± 0.02	8	0.27 ± 0.02	13	–	–	0.32 ± 0.05	4
35–37	0.43 ± 0.11	11	0.29 ± 0.01	13	0.51 ± 0.11	2	0.42 ± 0.10	14
38	0.67 ± 0.21	11	0.37 ± 0.05	4	0.43 ± 0.02	2	0.59 ± 0.05	3
39	1.02 ± 0.34	5	0.47 ± 0.08	2	0.66	1	–	–
40	0.98 ± 0.12	11	–	–	–	–	0.86 ± 0.15	4
41	1.01 ± 0.16	8	–	–	0.81 ± 0.34	2	0.69 ± 0.47	2
42	0.95 ± 0.11	4	–	–	–	–	–	–

3. Estriol

a) Normal Pregnancies

The first chemical studies showed that the estriol concentration is far higher in amniotic fluid than estrone and estradiol and that in contrast to these two estrogens up to a 100-fold increase occurred [104]. The data obtained at term in normal pregnancies are summarized in Table 52.

Measurements have been carried out as early as in the 9th–12th week of gestation [129, 198, 217–219]. Only a minor increase was found up to the 32nd week of gestation [217, 219–223] followed by an exponential rise toward term [224] or at least a rapid increase [217–219, 221, 225–228]. Beyond term most of the investigations described a decrease [220, 227, 229, 230] or a plateau [215, 221]. A further increase after 40 weeks of gestation has also been described [213]. Similar patterns were found when individual cases were monitored by repeated amniocenteses and determinations [125, 188, 220, 223]. Single determinations or serial measurements during the last 16 days before delivery indicate a tendency for a decrease of estriol in amniotic fluid but without statistical significance [231]. Length of labor, however, was correlated with estriol levels in amniotic fluid [231]. Using RIA

procedures for unconjugated estriol and immunoreactive estriol measurements in amniotic fluid [129], a decrease after term is obvious (Table 53).

Difference in amniotic fluid concentration between populations at sea level and high altitudes was found: 406 ± 49 and 323 ± 54 (SEM) μg/liter [236].

The published data indicate a wide range of values. To demonstrate the influence of gestational age and method of determination the values are grouped together in Table 54.

Table 52. Estriol in normal human amniotic fluid at term

Method	n	Estriol (μg/liter)			Ref.
		Free	Conjugated	Total	
Spectrophotometry	1	30.6	1892	–	104
Spectrophotometry	10	60.2	794	–	105
GLC	7	56.2	932	–	109
Spectrophotometry	–	16	616	–	232
Spectrophotometry	29	–	–	894	233
Spectrophotometry	6	–	–	783	107
Spectrophotometry	24	–	–	706	108
GLC	?	–	–	885–1470	81
GLC	27	–	–	979	110
GLC	pool	–	–	1572	57
Spectrophotometry	12	–	–	730	216
GLC	4	–	–	1352	217, 225
Spectrophotometry	22	–	–	911	218
GLC	15	–	–	1028	214
GLC	32	–	–	1010	234
Fluorimetry	7	9	880	810	235
Spectrophotometry	–	–	–	704	229
Spectrophotometry	33	–	–	1696	215
GLC	113	–	–	1230	215a
Spectrophotometry	24	–	–	1254	219
Fluorimetry	12	–	–	881	220
RIA	–	–	–	908	230
Spectrophotometry	48	–	–	943	226
Spectrophotometry	9	–	–	1090	203
RIA	37	7.8	–	777	228
RIA	16	17.3	–	–	164
Gas chromatography	20	–	834	–	73
Gas chromatography	pool	–	813	–	73

Table 53. Unconjugated and immunoreactive estriol in normal human amniotic fluid [129]

Weeks of gestation	Estriol (μg/liter; mean ± SEM)			
	Unconjugated	n	Immunoreactive	n
9–16	0.93 ± 0.09	11	5.2 ± 1.0	10
38	220.0	2	558.5	2
39	114.2 ± 71.2	3	271.3 ± 109.1	3
40	73.9 ± 32.0	9	274.7 ± 50.3	9
41	21.1 ± 3.9	3	193.1 ± 93.9	3
42	32.4 ± 9.3	6	211.0 ± 25.9	6

Table 54. Estriol in human amniotic fluid

Weeks of gestation	n	Type of estrogen measured	Estriol (µg/liter) Range	Mean	Ref.
15–25	5	Total E_3 (conjugates)	23– 35	31.5	105
31–35	2		88– 118	103	
Term	10		513–1079	794	
30–40	27	Total E_3	225–1238	674	184
Near term	27	Total E_3	185–2298	979	110
32	1	Total E_3	118	–	214
36–40	13		60–3441	1028	
12–20	4	Total E_3	147– 300	214	217, 225
21–30	5		300– 500	385	
31–38	18		300–1680	706	
39–40	14		550–2000	1382	
10–20	23	Total E_3		21	218
21–30	12			83	
31–38	9			198	
39–40	22			911	
16	1	Total E_3	–	3	224
18	11		5– 10	8.4	
20	9		7– 10	9.4	
21	3		–	10	
>37	27		416–2130	–	
20	4	Total E_3	5– 40	28	221
26–30	5		20– 240	100	
31–38	12		110– 810	334	
40	1		–	2130	
42–43	4		1190–1416	1582	
36	6	Total E_3	144– 956	564	215
37	7		377–2370	1916	
39	16		466–3790	1130	
40	33		211–3640	1696	
41	30		750–3370	1588	
42	9		263–2560	1147	
43	7		368–3160	1377	
37–40	7	Total E_3	416–1251	810	235
18–20	7	Total E_3	8– 93	42	237
39–40	7		240–3190	1434	
			95% confidence limit		
12–26	9	Total E_3	7– 66	36	219
27–28	5		14– 84	49	

Continued next page

Table 54 (continued)

Weeks of gestation	n	Type of estrogen measured	Estriol (μg/liter) Range	Mean	Ref.
29–30	7		18– 168	92	219
31–32	7		60– 211	135	
33–34	6		60– 288	174	
35–36	10		66– 482	274	
37–38	12		231–1456	843	
39–40	24		537–1971	1254	
26–27	4	Total E_3	88– 125	102	220
28–29	6		57– 112	88	
30–31	15		69– 251	136	
32–34	32		103– 557	231	
35	5		269– 565	320	
36–38	46		226– 915	483	
39–41	36		499–1297	844	
30–32	6	Total E_3	–	176	226
33–36	29		–	430	
37–41	48		–	943	
32–42	13	Total E_3	110– 650	–	238
32–42	13	Total unconjugated E_3	1.7– 22	–	
11–15	25	Total free immunoreactive estrogens	–	1.59	125
16–20	59		–	1.55	
21–25	14		–	1.63	
26–30	15		–	1.80	
31–35	32		–	2.39	
36–40	44		–	4.06	
35–37	11	Total estrogens	–	590	187
38–41	20		–	1890	
>42	12		–	1270	
37+40	2	Total estrogens	271 + 352	–	239
15–18	67	Unconjugated E_3		1.22	228
19–20	19			1.81	
29–32	10			3.85	
33–36	39			3.84	
37–40	37			7.82	
15–18	67	Total E_3		27.5	228
19–20	19			42.6	
29–32	10			215.3	
33–36	39			364.7	
37–40	37			777.2	

The ratio of unconjugated E_3 to total E_3 decreases significantly ($P < 0.001$) throughout gestation [228], which could be due to differences in the source of the amniotic fluid during gestation. The wider range of values and the rapid increase during the last trimester of unconjugated E_3 favors the measurement of total E_3 in amniotic fluid [228].

A significant correlation of amniotic fluid and urinary estriol concentration has been found: r = 0.69 [214]; r = 0.719 [234]; r = 0.56 [220]; r = 0.77 [227]; and r = 0.80 [425]. This was also found in pathologic conditions [240], while others were not able to establish such correlations [218, 224, 241, 242, 425]. A significant correlation ($P < 0.05$) was found for estriol in amniotic fluid with maternal serum estriol but not for total estrogens [238].

A statistically significant positive correlation between conjugated estriol and the total concentration of 16-OH-D and 16-Keto A was found both in normal pregnancies (r = 0.65, $P < 0.001$) and in pregnancies with intrauterine fetal growth retardation (r = 0.73; $P < 0.001$) [425].

Correlations were also found between estriol in amniotic fluid, and fetal weight up to 4,000 g [188, 215, 219, 227, 229, 241]. Others could not confirm this [224, 242]. Placental weight appeared to be proportional to the estriol concentration in amniotic fluid [215, 241], but significant correlations were absent [110, 188, 217, 220, 241]. Significant correlations of estriol with the amniotic fluid volume could not be established [110, 188, 214]. Sex differences are not obvious from unconjugated or total estriol concentration in amniotic fluid (Tables 55 and 56).

An interesting finding appears to be that the unconjugated estriol in amniotic fluid is higher in labor than in cases with cesarean section without labor [164].

Besides the wide range of estriol levels in amniotic fluid, estriol particularly

Table 55. Unconjugated estriol in human amniotic fluid (μg/liter; mean ± SEM) [260]

Weeks of gestation	Unconjugated estriol	
	Male fetus	Female fetus
8–11	0.46 ± 0.21	0.85 ± 0.33
12–15	0.49 ± 0.08	0.77 ± 0.09
16–20	1.27 ± 0.16	1.48 ± 0.13
32–40	49.27 ± 26.1	22.11 ± 7.6

Table 56. Total estriol in normal human amniotic fluid at term according to the sex of the fetus

Estriol (μg/liter)		Ref.
Male fetus	Female fetus	
992	792	233
425	434	106
1095	927	188

in the last trimester of pregnancy (see Table 53), it was found that in a case of premature rupture with daily measurement over a period of 18 h little variation in estriol concentration occurs; repeated sampling after surgical induction of labor also revealed little variation of the estriol content over periods of up to 8 h [243]. It could also be shown that storage at different temperatures over 9 weeks and filtration did not influence estriol measurement in amniotic fluid [244].

That methodological factors can contribute to the wide range of absolute values of estriol in amniotic fluid as listed in Table 53 was exemplified in a study comparing E_3 measurements in amniotic fluid in three laboratories. The results indicated that all three methods tend to place particular values in the same categories of high medium, and low levels, but there was a considerable discrepancy between the estriol values in individual cases [245].

b) Complicated Pregnancies

In contrast to other steroids in amniotic fluid, fairly large numbers of estriol values have been obtained in various pregnancy complications; in general, perinatal morbidity was associated with the estriol level in amniotic fluid being 3.9% of the mean normal level for the corresponding stage of gestation in retarded intrauterine growth, it was 69% and in healthy infants 107% of the normal mean level [240].

α) Death in Utero. Giraud et al. [241] reported four cases of intrauterine fetal death, one at 28 weeks with 88 μg/liter estriol, the second at 33 weeks of gestation with 76 μg/liter, the third with 54 μg/liter at 30 weeks of gestation, and in the fourth case 450 μg/liter were found at 37 weeks of gestation, but death occurred after several days. Low values were also reported by Jørgensen [240] when the amniotic fluid was not contaminated with meconium. In a case of intrauterine fetal death and severe Rh isoimmunization, the concentration of estriol was below 20 μg/liter and the amniotic fluid was nearly devoid of other steroids [184].

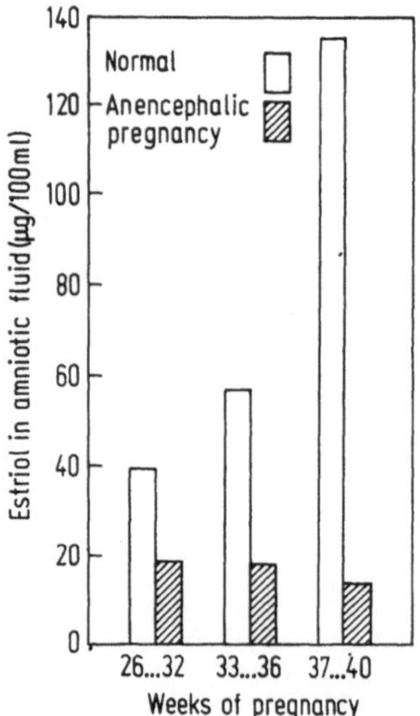

Fig. 12. The mean estriol concentration in normal pregnancy and in pregnancy with anencephalics. (Aleem et al. 1969 [217])

β) Anencephaly. In anencephaly, uniformly low estriol values have been found [73, 107, 108, 184, 188, 214, 217, 240]. From 26–40 weeks of gestation, low values of estriol and even a decrease could be observed in anencephaly (Fig. 12) [217]. In eight cases, Michie [107] not only determined very low estriol levels but also diminished estradiol and estrone concentrations. One case has been described with a normal level of estriol in the amniotic fluid [106]. Using the total estrogen measurement in another case, the value was in the lower range of normal [241].

γ) Preeclampsia—Renal Vascular Disease. In this complication of pregnancy, each author has investigated only a few cases, indicating that depending on the severity of the complication the estriol level in amniotic fluid could be normal or decreased [203, 214, 215, 217, 225, 241]. Recently, a larger number of cases could be studied by RIA at different times of gestation and various degrees of severity of clinical symptoms [129]. The data are shown in Table 57. Compared to the normal values (see Table 56), no definite deviations from the normal range are evident.

Table 57. Unconjugated and immunoreactive estriol in human amniotic fluid in patients with preeclampsia [129]

Clinical symptom	Weeks of gestation	Estriol (μg/liter; mean ± SEM)			
		Unconjugated	n	Immunoreactive	n
Edema	28–31	3.2 ± 0.4	7	35.9 ± 10.2	7
	32–34	2.8 ± 0.5	8	33.0 ± 7.5	8
	35–37	4.6 ± 1.5	11	55.7 ± 14.6	11
	38	6.0 ± 1.1	10	102.5 ± 28.7	10
	39	11.4 ± 5.4	4	159.3 ± 50.5	5
	40	31.4 ± 9.3	10	219.8 ± 34.8	10
	41	25.4 ± 9.4	7	211.4 ± 52.0	8
	42	20.0 ± 1.8	4	173.7 ± 9.1	4
Edema and proteinuria	28–31	6.5	1	40.6	1
	32–34	3.4	2	69.3	2
	35–37	–	–	–	–
	38	–	–	–	–
	39	64.6 ± 13.1	3	297,0 ± 36.8	3
	40	11.7	1	173.9	1
	41	21.1 ± 9.4	4	179.4 ± 56.7	4
	42	–	–	–	–

δ) Rh Isoimmunization. Nearly all investigators conclude from the data obtained that in pregnancy with severe Rh isoimmunization a low level of estriol is found in amniotic fluid [110, 129, 184, 188, 205, 214, 215, 217, 223, 235, 239, 246]. Unconjugated and immunoreactive estriol measurements showed low values in Rh disease [129] as shown in Table 58.

Others could only in part confirm this, demonstrating that in pregnancies terminating in abortion the amniotic fluid estriol values became low when serial measurements were carried out [128]. Later in pregnancy, only in some of the severely affected pregnancies were low levels measured [246]. Estriol conjugates were also found to be low in severe Rh incompatibility [235]. Dif-

Table 58. Unconjugated and immunoreactive estriol levels in human amniotic fluid in pregnancies complicated by Rh isoimmunization [129]

Weeks of gestation	n	Estril (μg/liter; mean ± SEM)	
		Unconjugated	Immunoreactive
28–31	10	3.0 ± 0.4	25.0 ± 4.2
32–34	13	2.4 ± 0.2	24.0 ± 3.1
35–37	13	3.0 ± 0.3	33.0 ± 6.7
38	4	3.3 ± 0.3	60.7 ± 8.1
39	2	4.5 ± 0.5	114.3 ± 25.1

Table 59. Unconjugated and immunoreactive estriol levels in human amniotic fluid in pregnancies complicated by diabetes mellitus

Weeks of gestation	n	Estriol (μg/liter; mean ± SEM)	
		Unconjugated	Immunoreactive
35–37	2	4.2 ± 1.2	83.5 ± 30.1
38	2	3.9 ± 1.0	154.7 ± 91.2
39	1	17.1	313.2
40	6	11.7 ± 8.9	156.4 ± 126.6

ferences in the conjugate ratio were noticed [247]. In mild Rh disease, the pattern and quantity of estriol conjugates did not differ significantly from normal [248]. It is obvious to differentiate between severely and mildly/moderately affected fetuses. In the latter group, the range of estriol values in amniotic fluid is similar to normal, and the increase during the course of pregnancy also demonstrates an identical pattern [184, 188, 212]. In individual cases, spectrophotometric results, therapeutic procedures, and estriol determinations with corresponding changes were observed [184, 188, 238].

The low estriol values in amniotic fluid in contrast to normal values in maternal blood and urine could reflect fetal renal failure. It was demonstrated [188, 223] that in severe Rh incompatibility low creatinine levels in amniotic fluid are found [249]. This might be due to the cardiovascular failure of the fetus and therefore failure to excrete normals amounts of creatinine into the amniotic fluid. By the same mechanisms low fetal excretion of estriol into the amniotic fluid might occur.

ε) Diabetes. Similar to the previously discussed complications, the severity of the abnormality appears to play a major role; however, from most of the data available, differentiation cannot be made. In severe cases, estriol appears to be low [164, 215, 225]. In others, differences to normal values could not be found [106, 110, 188, 215, 238, 241]. This applied to total estrogens and cortisol [238]. Table 59 summarizes recent results obtained by RIA [129].

Wide variability of the values and limited number of determinations do not permit a judgment when compared to the data of normal pregnancies.

ζ) Small-for-Date Infants. Various factors can be involved when intrauterine fetal hypotrophy occurs. Using fetal intrauterine growth as a common denominator, it could be demonstrated that significantly lower concentrations of estriol are present in amniotic fluid (Table 60). This was also found in another study, which shows that the average estriol level in the amniotic fluid of this group was 69% of the corresponding normal mean level [240].

Table 60. Estriol in human amniotic fluid in pregnancies with eutrophic and hypotrophic infants [226]

Weeks of gestation	Estriol (μg/liter; mean ± SD)				P[a]
	Eutrophic infants	n	Hypotrophic infants	n	
33–36	430.0 ± 191.7	29	185.7 ± 86.2	16	<0.001
37–41	943.8 ± 48.8		392.2 ± 258.9	27	<0.001

[a] P, Significance

Laatikainen and Peltonen [425] found that in three out of 12 cases with intrauterine fetal growth retardation the estriol level was below the 2.5 percentile obtained for the reference group, while maternal estriol levels were markedly decreased in 6 and slightly decreased in 5 more cases.

η) Polyhydramnios. Normal to low values have been reported in this condition, probably influenced by the extent of the polyhydramnios and the underlying cause of this deviation [110, 184, 215, 241].

θ) Postterm. In spite of some degree of uncertainty in establishing the exact time of confinement, it is obvious from the various reports that in pregnancies beyond 41 weeks of gestation there is a decrease of the estriol concentrations in amniotic fluid [187, 205, 215, 220, 229, 230, 241].

4. Estetrol

a) Normal Pregnancies

This steroid is mainly produced by the fetus and therefore represents a unique compound for the evaluation of the fetus [238]. This has been demonstrated for urine and serum measurements [250–252]. At term, the concentration was measured in pooled amniotic fluid and 83.6 μg/liter were found [57]. In 24 individual measurements of the steroid, a mean value of 99.7 ± 8.6 (SEM) μg/liter was determined [108]. Application of RIA in 14 samples of 13 third trimester patients revealed a range of 0.8–13 μg/liter for the unconjugated moiety [238]. Another group reported a single determination of 6 μg/liter at term [81].

b) Complicated Pregnancies

In a case of anencephaly, estetrol could not be detected [108]. In diabetes mellitus, no significant difference was found [238]. In Rh disease, this steroid indicated better correlation with the clinical status than unconjugated or total estriol in amniotic fluid [238].

F. Steroid Conjugates in Human Amniotic Fluid

Besides the free moiety of the steroid molecule, biologically steroid hormones are to a large extent cojugated as sulfate or glucuronide as a monoconjugate or as a double conjugate, such as disulfate or mixed conjugate. Sulfates represent mainly a transport form and glucuronides are suitable for excretion. In pregnancy and particularly in amniotic fluid, such conjugates play a part in three ways:

1) The type of conjugation depends on the sources of steroids in amniotic fluid.
2) The pattern of steroid conjugates is possibly influenced by differences in transfer and metabolism of estriol conjugates by the amniotic membranes.
3) The pattern of steroid conjugates might be influenced by various disturbances within the fetoplacental unit or in the maternal compartment.

According to the groups of steroids in the previous chapters, the type and quantity of the steroid conjugates in normal and abnormal pregnancies will be presented.

I. C_{30}, C_{29}, and C_{28} Steroids

For these steroids, no qualitative and quantitative data on conjugates have been found.

II. C_{27} Steroids

Although larger studies have been carried out mainly for cholesterol, there are no detailed studies regarding the type and extent of conjugation.

III. Δ^5-C_{21} Steroids

This group of steroids was only found as disulfates (see Sect. D. III) [59, 60, 103]. One of these compounds (pregn-5-ene-3β,20-diol) was quantitated in three pregnancies with anencephalic fetuses in the disulfate fraction (range 6–12 μg/liter). In normal amniotic fluid, a concentration of 22 μg/liter had been found [59, 103]. For 17α-hydroxypregnenolone, the free and sulfate fractions were quantitated, showing a preponderance of the latter [58].

IV. Δ^4-C_{21} Steroids

In 1968, free and conjugated cortisol and cortisone were reported, and the conjugate was considered to be a glucuronide [56]. Others have found cortisol and cortisone as sulfates and as free moiety [66, 67]. Similar findings were obtained for corticosterone and 11-dehydrocorticosterone. 11-Dehydrocorticosterone was only found as sulfate [66]. Recently, it was concluded from the available data that about 20% of the total cortisol is unconjugated in amniotic fluid [143] and that most of the corticoids are present as sulfates [253]. It is noteworthy that in anencephaly, unconjugated glucocorticoids were similar to normal pregnancy, but the conjugated form was low [253]. This discrepancy is explained by assumption that the conjugate is derived from the fetus while unconjugated cortisol might also be derived from the amniotic membranes [253].

A better correlation of glucocorticoid conjugates than of cortisol to fetal lung maturation was demonstrated [253], and further studies indicated that conjugated glucocorticoids had a better concurrence with the L/S ratio than cortisol [254].

V. 17-Hydroxycorticosteroids

These steroids are present in amniotic fluid as free moiety and as sulfates and glucuronides [66, 193, 194]. In Table 61, the data are listed according to weeks of gestation and sex of the fetus and clinical diagnosis.

No major changes were found corresponding to age of gestation or sex of the fetus. The lower concentration in anencephaly is obvious. A slightly different distribution was reported by Schweitzer et al. [66]. In a pool of amniotic fluid at term 10% were found in the free fraction, 67% as glucuronides, and 22% as sulfates. In the adrenalectomized patient, differences to

Table 61. 17-Hydroxycorticosteroids in human amniotic fluid

Clinical diagnosis and Weeks of gestation	Fetal sex	n	17-Hydroxycorticosteroids						Ref.
			Free		Glucuronide		Sulfates		
			μg/ml	%	μg/ml	%	μg/ml	%	
Normal, 26–36 weeks	Male and female	10 10	38.5 42.8	26.4 18.4	64.0 107.9	44.0 43.8	42.8 104.8	29.8 37.7	194
Normal, at term	Male Female	10	37.3	16.3	119.9	50.4	73.5	33.3	193
Anencephaly	Male and female	4	17.5	30.7	22.2	38.9	17.9	30.3	193
Adrenalectomized patient, 38 weeks		1	35.5	20.5	79.7	45.7	59.0	33.8	194

normal were not found [194]. Taking the amniotic fluid values published by Gadd [195] into account, Wade and Abramovich [193] found that the minimum and maximum 17-hydroxycorticosteroid contents of amniotic fluid in normal and anencephalic pregnancies do not differ as demonstrated in Table 62.

Such an approach, however, only appears to be valid when the actual amniotic fluid volume is known.

Table 62. Comparison of 17-hydroxycorticosteroid concentration in human amniotic fluid in normal and anencephalic pregnancies [193]

Clinical diagnosis	Amniotic fluid volume (ml)	17-Hydroxycorticosteroid (μg/liter)			
		Total	Free	Glucuronide	Sulfate
Normal	500	119.9	18.6	56.7	44.6
	1100	263.9	41.0	124.8	98.1
Anencephalic	2000	115.2	35.6	44.4	35.8
	6000	345.6	105.0	133.2	107.4

VI. Pregnane Steroids

Tetrahydrocortisol, tetrahydrocortisone, and tetrahydro-11-dehydrocorticosterone, 5β-pregnan-20-one-3α-ol, 5α-pregnan-20-one-3α,16α-diol, 5β-pregnane-20-one-3β, 16α-dione, 5β-pregnane-20-one-3α, 6α-diol, and 5α-pregnane-3β, 16α,20α-triol could only be found as glucuronides [66, 67, 72]. Pregnanetriol has been identified on the one hand as glucuronide [72] but on the other hand it was stated that it is normally present as sulfate; in abnormal pregnancies, it is also present in the free fraction [78].

As sulfate, the following pregnane steroids were found: 5α-pregnen-3β,20α-diol, 5α-pregnane-3β,20α-diol, 5α-pregnane-20-one-3α-21-tril, 5β-pregnane-20-one-3α,6α-diol, and 5α-pregnane-3α-20α,21-triol [59, 60, 76]. The major portion of pregnanediol is present in amniotic fluid as glucuronide [72] when compared to the values found for pregnanediol [57, 184]. Unconjugated pregnanediol was not found [75].

VII. Δ^5-C_{19} Steroids

The isomers androst-5-one-3β,17α-diol and androst-5-ene-3β,17β-diol as well as 16β-hydroxydehydroepiandrosterone are present in amniotic fluid as disulfates [76]. From the available data, it appears that most of the dehydroepiandrosterone in amniotic fluid is present as sulfate [57, 89, 178]. The 16-hydroxylated moiety, however, is only present in about 1/10 as disulfate and a small amount as monosulfate [57, 59]. Similar proportions seemed to be relevant for 16-keto-A [57, 59, 81]. Androst-5-ene-3β,16β-17α-triol has been found mainly in the disulfate form [60] and only a small quantity as glucuronide [72].

VIII. Δ^4-C_{19} Steroids

There are ample data to show that testosterone is present in unconjugated form in amniotic fluid (see Table 42). However, the steroid is also present as glucuronide and even a greater proportion is found as sulfate [94].

IX. 17-Ketosteroids

Similar to 17-hydroxycorticoids in human amniotic fluid, 17-ketosteroids were found in the free, glucuronide, and sulfate fractions as listed in Table 63. Differences are not discernable except for the low values in anencephaly.

Table 63. 17-Ketosteroids in human amniotic fluid [193, 194]

Clinical diagnosis and weeks of gestation	Fetal sex	n	17-Ketosteroids						Ref.
			Free		Glucuronide		Sulfate		
			mg/liter	%	mg/liter	%	mg/liter	%	
Normal/ abnormal, 26–36 weeks	Male and female	10	9.4	13.7	38.5	48.7	29.5	37.6	194
Normal, at term	Male	10	11.6	10.3	63.1	55.2	41.7	35.5	193
	Female	10	13.6	11.1	58.4	47.9	51.7	42.1	193
Anencephaly	Male and female	4	3.0	10.4	13.5	46.7	12.7	42.8	193
Adrenal- ectomized patient, 38 weeks	–	1	9.4	7.9	67.5	56.7	42.1	35.4	194

Table 64. Comparison of 17-ketosteroids in human amniotic fluid in normal and anencephalic pregnancies [193]

Clinical diagnosis	Amniotic fluid volume (ml)	17-Ketosteroids (mg/liter)			
		Total	Free	Glucuronide	Sulfate
Normal	500–1100	59.8	6.7	30.4	23.2
		131.6	13.7	66.8	51.1
Anencephaly	2000–6000	58.4	6.0	27.0	25.4
		175.2	18.6	81.0	76.2

Calculation of total amniotic fluid content in normal and anencephalic pregnancies according to the data of Gadd [195] revealed no differences (Table 64), but the validity of such an approach has to be questioned as previously indicated. The data are shown in Table 64.

X. Estrogens

The three major estrogens, estrone, estradiol and estriol, have been found as free, sulfate, and glucuronide conjugated moiety. The data in Table 65 were obtained by differential enzyme hydrolysis.

Table 65. Estrogens (μg/ml) in amniotic fluid after differential enzyme hydrolysis [22].

	Free	Glucuronide	Sulfate
Estrone	2	6	3
Estradiol-17β	3	4	2
Estriol	23	350	63

Up to 16 weeks of gestation, Klopper [255] found the following distribution for estriol in amniotic fluid: free = 16.4, glucuronide = 77.5, and sulfate = 41.3 μg/liter. Others have differentiated between free and conjugated forms or have compared the free portion to the total amount of the respective steroid as shown in Table 66 [104, 105, 109].

It is obvious that the only minor changes occur for estrone and estradiol during pregnancy regarding the relationship of free and conjugated moiety

Table 66. Free and conjugated estrogens in human amniotic fluid during gestation

Weeks of gestation	n	Estrone (μg/liter)			Estradiol-17β (μg/liter)			Estriol (μg/liter)			Ref.
		Free	Conjugated	Total	Free	Conjugated	Total	Free	Conjugated	Total	
16–20	2	0	3.1	–	0	0	–	6.2	19.4	–	104
40	1	26.5	0	–	13.5	0	–	30.6	1892.0	–	
At term	7	5.6	8.0	–							109
15–25	5	0.8	–	2.5	0.06	–	0.6	6.2	–	31.4	105
31–35	2	0.7	–	1.7	1.0	–	2.3	4.5	–	103.2	
At term	9/10	1.9	–	4.4	2.1	–	3.1	60.2	–	794	

Table 67. Levels of free and conjugated estrogens in human amniotic fluid at term [109]

Steroid	Free	Conjugate
Δ^{11}-Estradiol-17α	–	2.0
2-Methoxyestrone	+	+
16-Epiestriol	–	5.7
17-Epiestriol	+	1.9
16α-Hydroxyestrone	2.7	24.7
16β-Hydroxyestrone	–	17.8
160xo-estradiol	3.6	26.5
15α-Hydroxyestrone	1.0	5.5

+, Trace amount –, Not determined

and the total content. However, for estriol a 20–100-fold increase is found, and the conjugated fraction increases 10–30 times more than the free estriol portion. This is true for the glucuronide and sulfate fraction as well [223, 256]. Very limited data are available for other estrogens (Table 67).

Very detailed studies have been done with estriol. The distribution of the major conjugate fractions is shown in Table 68. The distribution of estriol conjugates (%) in human amniotic fluid is summarized in Table 69.

Table 68. Free and conjugated estriol in human amniotic fluid

Clinical diagnosis and weeks of gestation	Estriol conjugates (μg/liter)						Ref.
	Free estriol	E_3–16 Glucuronide	E_3–3 Glucuronide	E_3–3 Sulfate	E_3–3 Sulfate/ 16 Glucuronide	Sum of fractions	
Normal, 37–40 weeks	9	560	–	75	245	889	235
Severe Rh disease, 29–30 weeks	2.6	24.7	–	19.3	48.5	95.1	
Normal, 39–40 weeks	–	738	–	281	312	1443	237
Normal, 18–20 weeks	–	7.2	2.3	7.1	12.8	29.6	
At term	–	847	134	245	195	1420	248
Mild Rh disease	–	501	88	142	237	1010	
Normal, 32–40 weeks	–	31	53.8	114	198	–	247
Rh disease, 26–37 weeks	–	226	83.0	85.6	159	–	

Table 69. Distribution of estriol conjugates in human amniotic fluid

Clinical diagnosis and weeks of gestation	Estriol conjugates (%)				Ref.
	E_3–16 Glucuronide	E_3–3 Glucuronide	E_3–3 Sulfate	E_3–3 Sulfate/ 16 Glucuronide	
Normal, 37–40 weeks	61.1	–	9.0	28.9	235
Severe Rh disease, 29–30 weeks	24.8	–	22.0	50.5	
Normal, 39–40 weeks	51.0	9.0	19.0	21.0	237
Normal, 18–20 weeks	28.0	8.0	22.0	42.0	
At term	61.1	15.9	9.1	14.0	248
Mild Rh disease	53.3	15.1	9.4	22.3	
At term, normal	50.2	15.0	3.1	30.3	232

Although the determination of the estriol conjugates demonstrates in severe Rh disease a diminution compared to normal levels [235], which is not evident in mild involvement [248], it indicates that there is a change in the ratio of E_3-16 glucuronide to estriol-3-sulfate, 16-glucuronide [235, 247, 256]. A similar ratio is, however, also seen in early pregnancy with Rh disease [237]. However, at a comparable age of gestation, this difference is normal, and Rh-induced changes are very obvious [247], possibly reflecting a regression toward a metabolic pattern of early gestation. Two more sulfate conjugates of estriol were isolated and quantitated in amniotic fluid, but have also been found in umbilical cord and maternal serum [257]. At term, these two conjugates were found in the concentrations shown in Table 70.

Table 70. Estriol-16-sulfate and estriol-3,16-disulfate in human amniotic fluid, umbilical cord blood, and maternal blood [257]

	Total estriol (μg/liter)	Estriol-16-sulfate (μg/liter)	Estriol-3,16-disulfate (μg/liter)
Amniotic fluid	2022	2.7	3.8
Umbilical cord blood	2496	0.5	11.9
Maternal blood	296	0.6	1.1

Recently, an extensive study on E_3-3-glucuronide (E_3-3-G) and E_3-16-glucuronide (E_3-16-G) in amniotic fluid during normal pregnancy was published [258]. At 16 weeks of gestation, E_3-3-G and E_3-16-G were present in amniotic fluid in similar mean concentrations (5 ng/ml). The concentrations of both steroid conjugates increased as pregnancy progressed and reached a mean of 300 ng/ml for E_3-3-G and 1,150 ng/ml for E_3-16-G at 40 weeks of gestation. Fetal sex differences could not be detected, and significant correlations could not be found for birth weight and placental weight. The measurement of E_3-16-G could be used as an additional test for assessing fetal lung maturity. The authors proposed the following classification: up to 600 ng/ml = immature, 600–1,000 ng/ml = borderline and above 1,000 ng/ml = mature [258].

G. Steroid Profiles in Human Amniotic Fluid and Distribution of Steroids in Several Compartments

Simultaneous measurements of various steroids in amniotic fluid have been carried out to a limited extent. For C_{30}, C_{29}, C_{28}, and C_{27} steroids, it was found that they represent about 2% of the total sterol content in human amniotic fluid and that about 10%–20% consist of cholestanol and cholesterol precursors [53]. The distribution of steroids (%) in various compartments and fetal substances is summarized in Table 71.

Table 71. Distribution of steroids (%) in vernix caseosa, meconium, amniotic fluid, placenta, and maternal serum [53]

Sterols	Vernix caseosa	Meconium	Amniotic fluid	Placenta	Maternal serum
Cholesterol	78.87	85.02	90.39	98.97	99.03
Cholestanol	1.71	2.37	1.41	0.71	0.03
Δ^7-Cholestenol	17.01	9.58	5.74	0.03	0.03
7-Dehydrocholesterol	0.14	0.34	0.36	0.14	0.19
[a]-Cholesterol	0.04	0.20	0.07	0.03	0.02
Desmosterol	0.08	0.56	0.09	0.04	0.04
Methyl sterols	2.11	1.89	1.91	0.05	0.03

[a] An unlocated double bond

Table 72. Comparison between cholesterol concentration in human amniotic fluid, maternal vein blood, and umbilical cord blood in 80 cases [115]

	Cholesterol (mg/100 ml; mean ± SEM)
Amniotic fluid	11.7 ± 0.9
Umbilical cord blood	84.8 ± 1.7
Maternal vein blood	269.0 ± 6.1

Absolute amounts of cholesterol have recently been compared in amniotic fluid and maternal and umbilical cord blood at term [115] as shown in Table 72. There was a lack of correlation between cholesterol levels in amniotic fluid, maternal blood, and umbilical cord blood and fetal weight [115]. Lack of correlation of cholesterol in maternal serum and amniotic fluid was also reported by others [116].

C_{21} steroids were simultaneously quantitated by some investigators [66, 67]. The data are shown in Table 73.

Table 73. Some C_{21} steroids simultaneously determined in human amniotic fluid

Steroid (μg/100 ml)											Type of sample	Ref.
Cortisol	Cortisol sulfate	Cortisone	Cortison sulfate	Corticosterone	Corticosterone sulfate	11-Dehydrocorticosterone	11-Dehydrocorticosterone sulfate	11-Deoxycorticosterone sulfate	Tetrahydrocortisol glucuronide	Tetra hydrocortisone glucuronide		
1.8	3.0	1.1	3.1	0.1	4.8	0.1	1.8	0.7	2.3	12.3	Pool	66
–	3.4	–	2.6	–	4.0	–	–	–	–	–	Single samples (n = 10)	66
2.0	3.6	1.6	2.9	0.2	3.8	–	–	–	2.2	11.7	Single samples (n = 8)	67

The pattern and the quantitative relationship between the sulfates and glucuronides closely resemble the findings obtained from newborn urine [67, 259]. Different profiles are found in umbilical cord blood and maternal vein blood as listed in Table 74 [67].

The concentrations of the sulfates of cortisol, cortisone, and corticosterone decrease in magnitude from amniotic fluid to umbilical cord blood to maternal vein blood. This indicates that the fetal compartment is the main source of these conjugates and that the profiles in umbilical cord blood and maternal

Table 74. 17-Hydroxy- and 17-deoxycorticosteroid profiles in amniotic fluid, umbilical cord blood, and maternal vein blood [67]

Steroid	Amniotic fluid (μg/100 ml)	Umbilical cord blood (μg/100 ml)	Maternal vein blood (μg/100 ml)
Cortisol	2.0	3.1	25.5
Cortisol sulfate	3.6	1.3	0.2
Cortisone	1.6	8.5	7.3
Cortisone sulfate	2.9	0.5	0.0
Corticosterone	0.2	0.2	0.8
Corticosterone sulfate	3.8	2.7	0.2
Tetrahydro-cortisol glucuronide	2.2	2.3	1.9
Tetrahydro-cortisone glucuronide	11.7	4.1	1.6
Tetrahydro-11-dehydrocortico-sterone glucuronide	2.1	4.8	0.1

Table 75. Cortisol in premature and term deliveries [140]

	Cortisol (μg/100 ml; mean ± SD)					
	Spontaneous labor	n	Induced labor	n	Cesarean section	n
Term deliveries						
Cord blood	8.9 ± 5.0	14	6.2	2	4.3 ± 1.8	8
Maternal blood	53.5 ± 20.6	13	51.9 ± 16.6	4	70.1 ± 23.9	8
Amniotic fluid	5.3 ± 2.6	12	2.6 ± 0.6	4	2.4 ± 0.8	9
Premature deliveries						
Cord blood	5.2 ± 4.8	6	–	–	4.2 ± 2.5	6
Maternal blood	56.6 ± 16.9	5	–	–	71.0 ± 33.4	5
Amniotic fluid	3.5 ± 1.0	6	–	–	2.3	3

vein blood represent secretory and metabolic processes taking place in these compartments [67]. The change in relationship of cortisol and cortisone in the three compartments has also been confirmed by others [151]. A correlation exists between the cortisol concentration in amniotic fluid and umbilical cord blood [140, 144, 151], which was found to be significant ($P < 0.01$). Such close correlation could not be established between cortisol in amniotic fluid and maternal vein blood [144, 149, 156]. Comparison of the cortisol concentration in cord blood, maternal blood, and amniotic fluid in term and premature deliveries is shown in Table 75.

In a recent detailed study, the profile of corticosteroids in the maternal and fetal compartments were studied at term [424]. The data are summarized in Table 76.

These results indicate that the source of corticosteroid sulfates in amniotic fluid is mainly the fetal urine. The free corticosteroids seem to be derived from various sources and are subjected to interconversion. Changes of cortisol

Table 76. Concentration of corticosteroids in the maternal and fetal compartment in nine normal pregnancies at term [424]

	Steroid (μg/ml; mean ± SEM)			
	Cortisol	Cortisone	Cortisol sulfate	Corticosterone sulfate
Maternal peripheral blood	423.1 ± 69.9	42.2 ± 9.7	21.1 ± 3.2	16.0 ± 3.2
Umbilical artery	25.0 ± 4.1	47.2 ± 9.2	7.2 ± 1.0	32.5 ± 4.6
Umbilical vein	18.1 ± 3.1	47.8 ± 5.5	6.4 ± 1.5	30.6 ± 3.6
Newborn urine	18.6 ± 2.8	68.5 ± 12.5	173.5 ± 59.3	275.6 ± 72.2
Amniotic fluid	16.2 ± 2.2	9.0 ± 1.1	28.6 ± 5.0	35.2 ± 5.8
Fetal pulmonary fluid	22.3 ± 4.1	10.6 ± 1.7	37.4 ± 5.8	44.5 ± 8.3

Table 77. Cortisol and cortisone (ng/ml) in human amniotic fluid and umbilical cord blood [271]

Weeks of gestation	Amniotic fluid		Cord arterial blood		Cord venous blood	
	Cortisol	Cortisone	Cortisol	Cortisone	Cortisol	Cortisone
11–16	3.0	9.2	12.2	32.5	6.5	52.3
17–22	4.7	6.7	6.7	17.3	3.7	20.7
25–30	9.4	5.1	–	–	–	–
36–40[a]	18.0	10.6	36.0	62.6	20.5	70.5
36–40[b]	28.5	18.9	120.0	108.0	98.0	143.0
35[c]	24.7	28.0	15.6	80.0	39.7	163.0

[a] No labor
[b] Spontaneous labor
[c] Anencephaly

and cortisone during gestation in amniotic fluid and fetal blood are listed in Table 77, and for comparison two cases with anencephaly are included [271].

For progesterone a comparison of various compartments was done by Harbert et al. [122] as shown in Table 78.

Comparative data on 17α-OH pregnenolone are available in amniotic fluid and maternal serum [58] as listed in Table 79.

The profiles of 21-hydroxylated disulfate steroids are as follows [60]: 21-hydroxypregnenolone = 122 μg/liter, 3α,21-dihydroxy-5α-pregnane-20-one = 18 μg/liter, 5-pregnene-3β,20α,21-triol = 12 μg/liter, and trace amounts of 5α-pregnane-3α,20α,21-triol. The latter compound was found in amniotic

Table 78. Progesterone concentration in maternal and fetal plasma and amniotic fluid [122]

Source	n	Progesterone (μg/liter; mean ± SEM)
Maternal artery	37	160 ± 15
Maternal vein	50	150 ± 12
Placental pool	27	767 ± 81
Umbilical vein	49	724 ± 42
Umbilical artery	32	436 ± 58
Amniotic fluid	14	59 ± 20

Table 79. Concentration of unconjugated and sulfoconjugated 17α-OH pregnenolone (μg/liter; mean ± SEM) [58]

Clinical diagnosis	Amniotic fluid		Maternal plasma	
	Unconjugated	Sulfoconjugated	Unconjugated	Sulfoconjugated
Midpregnancy	1.5 ± 0.3	2.0 ± 0.2	0.9 ± 0.1	2.4 ± 0.5
Term. pregnancy not in labor	0.8 ± 0.1	3.6 ± 0.7	1.2 ± 0.2	2.1 ± 0.4
At delivery	0.8 ± 0.1	6.4 ± 0.7	3.2 ± 0.7	4.2 ± 0.6

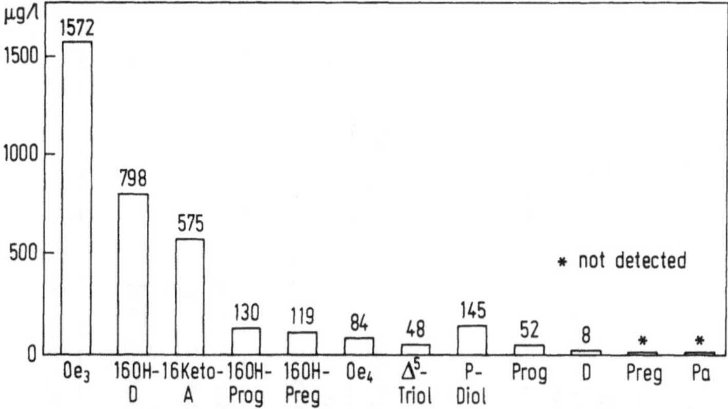

Fig. 13. Steroid profile obtained from a pool of normal human amniotic fluid at term. (Schindler et al. 1974 [260])

Table 80. Steroid disulfate profiles (μg/liter) in human amniotic fluid

Clinical diagnosis	5α-Pregnane-3α, 20α-diol	5α-Pregnane-3β, 20α-diol	5β-Pregnane-3α, 20α-diol	5-Pregnene-3β, 20α-diol	5-Pregnene-3β, 17α, 20α-triol	5-Androstene-3β, 17α-diol	5-Androstene-3β, 17β-diol	16α-OH DHEA	16β-OH DHEA	16-Keto-A	Ref.
12–17 weeks of gestation	7.1	4.9	11.9	4.0	–	6.3	2.6	8.2	2.3	15.0	76
At term	36.0	49.0	–	29.0	36.0	236.0	56.0	46.0	5.0	62.0	60
At term	–	38.0	–	22.0	26.0	224.0	42.0	48.0	88.0	6.0	59
Anencephaly (n = 27)	56.7	42.0	18.3	12.6	–	5.6	4.0	–	–	–	103

Table 81. Steroid profile (μg/liter) in normal human amniotic fluid at term and in anencephaly [108]

Clinical diagnosis	Total estrogens	Estriol	Estetrol	Estradiol	Estrone	16-Oxy-Δ^5-steroids	Δ^5-tiol	16-OHD 16-Keto-A	6β-OH Cortisol	6β-20-Dihydroxy-cortisol	6β-20-Dihydroxy-cortisone
Normal, at term	906.8	706.9	99.7	51.5	48.5	396.1	100.2	215.1	72.5	76.4	66.2
n	24	24	24	24	24	11	11	11	18	17	17
Anencephaly (n = 1)	144	144	ND[a]	ND	ND	2.5	ND	2.5	0.1	ND	ND

[a] ND, not detected

fluid with an anencephalic fetus in a concentration of 9.6 μg/liter, indicating that in anencephaly these steroid metabolites are mainly derived from the placenta and are present in normal concentrations.

Several studies have obtained data on steroid profiles of C_{21} and C_{19} steroids related to disulfates [59, 60, 76, 103]. The data are compiled in Table 80. Besides the increase throughout gestation, the data clearly demonstrated that these steroids derived mainly from placental sources are normal, while those depending on fetal adrenal secretion are low in anencephaly.

A number of studies have presented steroid profiles including C_{21}, C_{19}, and C_{18} steroids of placental and fetoplacental origin [57, 108, 184, 188, 260]. Such a profile is shown in Fig. 13.

Drafta et al. [108] have obtained a steroid profile as shown in Table 81 and compared these data to the profile in a pregnancy with anencephaly.

During the last trimester of pregnancy steroid profiles were obtained in normal and complicated pregnancies. The data are presented in Table 82.

Table 82. Steroid profiles (μg/liter) in human amniotic fluid during the last trimester in normal and complicated pregnancies [184, 188]

Clinical diagnosis	Dehydroepi-androsterone	Pregnanediol	16-Keto-A	16OH-D	Estriol
Normal last trimester	7.0 (n = 14)	164.3 (n = 29)	210.9 (n = 13)	599.6 (n = 18)	674.1
Diabetes mellitus[a]	2.3	174.0	94.0	145.0	427
Polyhydramnios[a]	5.5	197.0	34.0	80.0	154
Severe Rh isoimmunization[b]	4.5	224.0	ND[c]	ND	31.7
Severe Rh isoimmunization and intrauterine fetal death[a]	ND	6.0	ND	ND	<20.0
Anencephaly and intrauterine fetal death[a]	5.0	232.0	ND	ND	8.0

[a] n = 1
[b] n = 4
[c] ND, not detected

It is obvious that 16-hydroxylated steroids are diminished in severe Rh isoimmunization and anencephaly, and after longer standing intrauterine fetal death the amniotic fluid is nearly devoid of all steroids. Similar results were also obtained by others [205] as shown in Table 83. An increase in the various steroids during the last trimester toward term is seen.

In cases with congenital adrenal hyperplasia of the fetus, hydatidiform degeneration of the placenta [87], or placental sulfatase deficiency [82],

Table 83. Steroid profile (μg/liter) in human amniotic fluid of complicated pregnancies [205]

Clinical diagnosis and weeks of gestation	Estriol	16-Keto-A	16α-OH-D	n
Fetus not affected by Rh isoimmunozation, 32–36 weeks	287	126	246	6[a]
Fetus moderately to severely affected by Rh isoimmunization, 32–36 weeks	184	ND	24.6	8
Over term, 41 weeks	1590	366	715	5
Over term, 43 weeks	1100	185	418	2

[a] Estriol : n = 8

Table 84. Amniotic fluid steroid profile in a pregnancy with congenital adrenal hyperplasia of the fetus and a pregnancy with hydatidiform degeneration of the placenta (ng/ml) [82]

Type of pregnancy	Weeks of gestation	Testo-sterone	Andro-stene-dione	DHT	Estra-diol	Proge-sterone	17 α-OH Proge-sterone
Congenital adrenal hyperplasia	14	0.220	0.345	0.026	0.106	15	8.23
	22	0.606	1.224	–	0.067	15	20.68
	28	0.251	0.826	0.040	0.046	20	2.93
	34	0.200	–	–	–	–	3.67
Hydatidiform degeneration of the placenta	–	0.129	0.482	0.050	0.466	160	6.24
Controls[a] Male (n = 51)	–	0.188 ±0.014	0.348 ±0.032	0.024 ±0.003	0.036 ±0.009	34.7 ± 4.1	1.62 ±0.15
Female (n = 50)		0.022 ±0.002	0.156 ±0.029	0.024 –[b]	0.048 ±0.009	30.1 ± 0.4	1.51 ±0.10

[a] Mean values ± SEM
[b] Undetectable

Table 85. Steroid sulfate concentrations in human amniotic fluid (ng/ml) [82]

Steroid sulfate	Placental sulfatase defiency[a]	Normal amniotic fluid (1 liter pool)
D	30 (10–6610)	10
16α-OH-D	450 (30–7750)	160
16β-OH-D	Not determined	30
16-O-androstenediol 15β- 16-dihy-droxy-D	180 (10–4720)	40
A-triol	120 (10–5520)	30
16α-OH-Prog	250 (10–30130)	70
16, 18 dihydroxy-D	190 (10–3520)	40

[a] n = 3

steroid profiles have been measured in amniotic fluid as shown in Table 84.

It is obvious that 17α-OH-progesterone is elevated in all samples from pregnancies with pathologic conditions compared to normal controls. In a case with trisomy 21, the steroid levels in the amniotic fluid were found to be within the normal range [87].

A steroid profile of 16-hydroxylated C_{21} and C_{19} steroids in three cases of placental sulfatase deficiency compared to normal amniotic fluid [82] is presented in Table 85.

A comparison of nine normal pregnancies to nine pregnancies complicated by preeclampsia resulted in decreased estrogen and increased androgen levels in the amniotic fluid from the pathological cases [203] (Table 86).

Table 86. Steroid profile in amniotic fluid from nine normal pregnancies and nine pregnancies complicated by preeclampsia (ng/ml) [209]

Steroid	Normal pregnancies	Preeclampsia
Estrone	7	4.5
Estradiol	31	27
Estriol	1090	960
16-OHD	119	345
Androstenedione	9	17
Androstenediol	56	103

Comparison of steroid hormone profiles of one and two steroids in various compartments have been done by several investigators as total, free, or unconjugated moieties [66, 82, 109, 164, 188, 222, 223, 255, 257, 260]. It was demonstrated that on the one hand the profiles in cord blood and maternal blood are quite different from amniotic fluid from a quantitative point of view

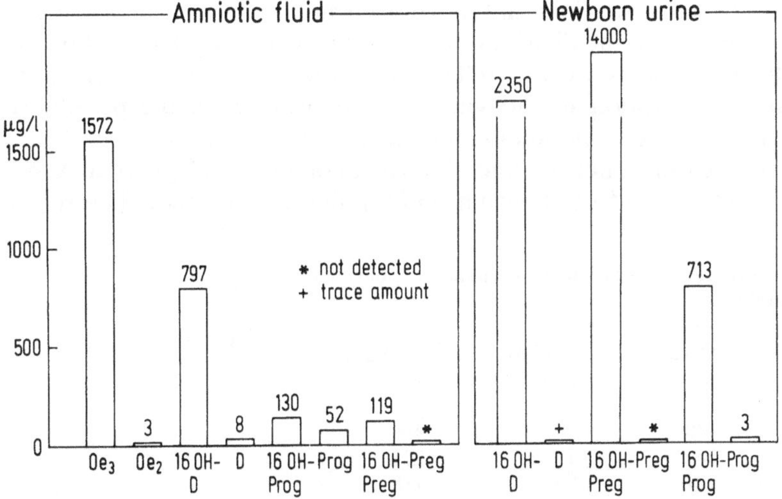

Fig. 14. Comparison of steroid pairs in amniotic fluid and newborn urine. (Schindler et al. 1974 [260])

[188, 260], but there is a close relationship between fetal and newborn urine [66, 119, 260]. This is also true when the free and conjugated forms of estriol are considered [222, 255]. Estriol is present mainly as glucuronide, and an equal level of sulfates is found in both biologic fluids [222]. Comparison to the cord blood demonstrates the preponderance of sulfates in this compartment [222]. A comparison of steroid pairs in amniotic fluid and newborn urine is shown in Fig. 14.

Data on the distribution of free and conjugated estrogens in cord plasma, amniotic fluid, and maternal blood are shown in Table 87.

Table 87. Estrogens (μg/liter) in cord plasma, amniotic fluid, and maternal plasma at term [109]

Estrogen	Cord plasma		Amniotic fluid		Maternal plasma	
	Free	Conjugated	Free	Conjugated	Free	Conjugated
Estriol	137	1260	56.2	932	6.5	124
Estradiol-17β	7.4	3.4	+	1.4	19.0	4.4
Estrone	24.3	26.2	5.6	8.0	11.1	79.2
$^{11}E_2$ 17α	–	2.2	–	2.0	–	1.4
2 ME E_1	1.4	2.8	+	+	2.2	2.1
16 Epi-E_3	1.7	5.4	–	5.7	+	6.3
17 Epi-E_3	+	1.0	+	1.9	–	–
16 OH E_1	2.6	46.6	2.7	24.7	0.8	27.0
16β-OH E_1	1.4	9.3	–	17.8	–	4.1
15α-OH E_1	2.7	5.5	1.0	5.5	+	3.4
160xo E_2	3.4	60.7	3.6	26.5	0.9	15.5

+, Trace amount –, Not detected

For estriol, a similar distribution in cord plasma and amniotic fluid was found by others [232]. In addition, comparison to newborn urine was carried out as listed in Table 88. These data again demonstrate the similarity of estriol moieties in amniotic fluid and newborn urine.

In another study [257], the distribution of total estriol, estriol-16-sulfate and estriol-3-16-disulfate was compared in the same three compartments (Table 89).

Changes in concentration in the various compartments show parallelism [223, 238, 164], and the correlation can be significant [214, 234].

Unconjugated estriol in normal and abnormal conditions of pregnancy was measured in maternal and cord serum and amniotic fluid [164]. The results

Table 88. Estriol (μg/liter) in cord plasma, amniotic fluid, and newborn urine [168]

Estriol	Cord plasma	Amniotic fluid	Newborn urine
Free	49	16	196
Conjugated	360	616	1271
"Sulfate"-fraction	227	70	118
"Glucuronide"-fraction	38	386	979

are compiled in Table 90. A similar study was done for unconjugated cortisol [164]. The results are listed in Table 91.

Both tables illustrate that unconjugated E_3 and cortisol in amniotic fluid undergo similar changes. Labor raises the steroid content. Pathologic conditions of pregnancy, such as diabetes, decrease these steroid levels in amniotic fluid.

A detailed study on C_{21} and C_{18} steroid sulfates in placental sulfatase deficiency compared steroid profiles in maternal plasma, cord plasma, and

Table 89. Concentration of total estriol, estriol-3-sulfate and estriol-3,16-disulfate (μg/liter) in cord plasma, amniotic fluid, and maternal plasma in five cases [257]

	Cord plasma	Amniotic fluid	Maternal plasma
Total estriol	2496	2022	296
Estriol-3-sulfate	0.5	2.7	0.6
Estriol-3,16-disulfate	11.9	3.8	1.1

Table 90. Unconjugated estriol in maternal and cord serum and amniotic fluid in normal and abnormal pregnancies (ng/ml; mean ± SEM) [164]

Clinical diagnosis	Unconjugated estriol (ng/ml; mean ± SEM)					
	Maternal serum	n	Cord serum	n	Amniotic fluid	n
Not in labor (cesarean section)	11.0 ± 1.12	16	87.32 ± 17.55	16	17.30 ± 5.66	16
Labor	15.48 ± 1.17	14	137.66 ± 26.13	14	43.81 ± 9.54	14
Normal	13.26 ± 0.91	30	110.81 ± 15.8	30	30.55 ± 6.19	20
Diabetes	11.87 ± 1.76	9	80.87 ± 23.1	9	12.78 ± 4.58	6
Stress	6.18 ± 1.2	8	57.29 ± 14.07	8	19.68 ± 11.2	5

Table 91. Unconjugated cortisol in amniotic fluid in maternal and cord serum and amniotic fluid in normal and abnormal pregnancies [164]

Clinical diagnosis	Unconjugated cortisol (μg/100 ml; mean ± SEM)					
	Maternal serum	n	Cord serum	n	Amniotic fluid	n
Not in labor (cesarean section)	32.46 ± 2.29	16	22.14 ± 1.76	16	5.69 ± 1.26	10
Labor	43.14 ± 3.34	14	33.07 ± 2.78	10	7.8 ± 0.68	16
Normal	37.44 ± 2.18	30	27.24 ± 1.87	30	6.94 ± 6.74	19
Diabetes	43.17 ± 10.62	9	28.16 ± 4.15	9	6.05 ± 1.17	6
Stress	28.8 ± 4.19	8	35.44 ± 4.4	8	12.02 ± 2.4	5

amniotic fluid. In the latter two instances, normal values could be included for comparison to pregnancies with placental sulfatase deficiency [82] (Table 92).

Table 92. Steroid sulfates (ng/ml) in maternal plasma, umbilical vein plasma, and amniotic fluid in placental sulfatase deficiency (PSD) [82]

Steroid	Maternal plasma	Cord plasma		Amniotic fluid	
	(n = 1)	PSD (n = 4)	Control (n = 4)	PSD (n = 3)	Control (1 liter pool)
D	760	390	260	30	20
16-OHD	13080	1860	1050	450	160
16β-OH-D	2130	590	230	ND[a]	30
16-Keto-A					
15β,16-Dihydroxy-D	610	410	120	180	40
16, 18 Dihydroxy-D	2190	130	190	190	40
A-triol	900	310	100	120	30
16-OH-preg	3180	630	230	250	70

[a] ND, not detected

H. Transfer and Metabolism of Steroids in Human Amniotic Membranes

It was shown in the previous chapter that steroids are present in amniotic fluid in the free form and as various conjugated moieties. The question arises as to whether these steroids pass through the amniotic membranes to the maternal compartment or if steroids are also transferred from the maternal compartment into the amniotic fluid via the amniotic membranes.

After bolus injection of radioactive cortisol into the maternal circulation, radioactivity was found in the fetal plasma but not in the amniotic fluid, leading to the conclusion that the transfer was via the placenta and no radioactivity passes through the amniotic membranes into the amniotic fluid [261]. Others injected radioactive dehydroepiandrosterone into the uterine artery 15 min before interruption of pregnancy and found radioactivity subsequently in the fetus but not in the amniotic fluid [262]. Using a continuous infusion technique into the mother with tritiated cortisol for 4–5 h, radioactivity was present not only in the fetal circulation but also in fetal urine and amniotic fluid [206]. In fetal urine, more than half of the activity was in the conjugate fraction, suggesting that most of the conjugated steroids found in the amniotic fluid are dependent on fetal voiding, while free steroids may enter the amniotic fluid by other pathways, such as the fetal surface of the placenta or via chorion and amnion [206].

Regarding the amniotic cavity, several studies have been done to elucidate the pathways of steroids from the amniotic fluid. Unconjugated estrogens disappear rapidly from amniotic fluid and can be found in fetal tissues, placenta, and maternal urine [262, 263]. Studies with labeled estrone sulfate and free estriol indicate a tenfold greater transfer of unconjugated hormones [264]. In contrast to fetal skin, where most of the steroids were present as sulfates, the steroids in the fetal membranes were present in the unconjugated form. Further studies have elucidated this point. It could be demonstrated by dialysis experiments that estriol transverses the amnion at about twice the rate of either the sulfate or the glucuronide [265, 266]. The transfer across the chorion is less rapid than through the amnion for all compounds, However, hydrolysis of the sulfates occurs in the chorion [265–267], and sulfatase activity is found in the amnion [265–267]. Hydrolysis of the glucuronides could not be detected [266].

Therefore, hydrolysis of the steroid sulfates by the chorion facilitates transfer to the mother. Glucuronides are poorly transferred and not hydrolyzed by the membranes [266]. The more rapid transfer of sulfates compared to glucuronides from the amniotic cavity to the maternal compartment and hydrolysis of sulfates by the fetal membranes were also verified by others [268].

Transfer will certainly also depend on gradients within the tissues and among the compartments as well as on binding. Indeed, a progesterone gradient has been found in the fetal membranes [130] comparing tissue near the placenta and distant fetal membrane regions, resulting in mean values of 85.7 and 60.8 μg/100 g, respectively ($P < 0.005$). This also demonstrates that progesterone concentration in the fetal membranes is higher than in the uterine vein blood, which drains the placenta with 56.3 μg/100 ml [269] or 47.3 μg/100 ml [270], and also higher than in amniotic fluid with 2–5 μg/100 ml [99, 125, 126, 188, 271], demonstrating tissue and compartment gradients. Therefore, specific binding needs to be present, Indeed, such binding was demonstrated in human fetal membranes, but not due to transcortin, a progesterone receptor or a glucucorticoid receptor [272]. The demonstration of a unique protein with high affinity for progesterone that appears in the fetal membranes before but near the onset of parturition explains the findings of Pulkkinen and Enkola [130] and may act by progesterone withdrawl in combination with continued estrogen stimulation on the mechanism of induction of labor [272]. Therefore, three processes regarding steroids do occur in the fetal membranes:

1) Binding of steroids
2) Hydrolysis of steroids (conjugation has not been demonstrated)
3) Metabolism of steroids

The last point can be differentiated into the capacity to synthesize and to metabolize steroids. Only few studies have been carried out so far. Synthesis of cortisol was recently reported [271]. There is also evidence that chorion laeve is capable of progesterone synthesis from pregnenolone, but not from cholesterol as substrate [272]. Chorion laeve from term and early gestation did not show differences. Progesterone formation by the amnion could not be demonstrated [272].

Metabolism of steroids by fetal membranes has been investigated mainly concerning progesterone and C_{19} steroids. However, some studies have been done on corticosteroid metabolism by amniotic membranes [47, 271, 271a, 271b].

In contrast to the metabolic activity of the placenta and fetal tissues converting cortisol to cortisone, it was shown that the amniotic membranes (mainly chorion) convert cortisone to cortisol [271, 271a]. This metabolic event increases with gestational age. High values were found after 16 weeks of gestation until after labor had started. Thereafter, a rapid decrease was noted [271]. Similar findings were reported by others [271a]. The reverse reaction was consistently lower, averaging 65% for placental metabolism of cortisone to cortisol and 10.2% for chorionic cortisol to cortisone conversion [271]. By this, a net gain of the active hormone cortisol results from the bidirectional interconversion of cortisol and cortisone in amniotic membranes reaching 40%–50% by term [271a]. Studies on the ability of the amniotic membranes to convert cortisone to cortisol showed significant differences ($P < 0.001$) comparing pregnancies with infants developing respiratory distress syndrom and a control group [271b]. In addition, it was observed that when labor commences with spontaneous membrane rupture there is a significantly greater net production of cortisol by the membrane than if labor begins with contractions or bleeding ($P < 0.001$) [271b]. These findings are in good agreement with the high cortisol/cortisone ratio in amniotic fluid [271, 424], which rises with gestational age [152].

Recently, the in vitro conversion of pregnenolone to progesterone by term human fetal membranes was studied [273]. The data are listed in Table 93.

Table 93. Conversion of pregnenolone to progesterone (n mol/min/g tissue) by homogenates of human fetal membranes at term (38–40 weeks)

Type of tissue	After labor	n	Prior to labor (elective cesarean section)	n
Chorion (pars reflexa)	21.8 ± 2.1[a]	10	15. ± 2.0	18
Amnion (pars reflexa)	0.2, 0.5, 0.5, 0.8, 2.5, ND[b]	8	ND	18
Amnion (pars placentaris)	0.12, ND[c]	12	ND	18

[a] Mean ± SD
[b] Not detected in 3 cases
[c] Not detected in 11 cases

The results point toward the possibility that during labor steroid metabolism in fetal membrane might be activated [273].

Regarding progesterone, incubation studies with amnion and chorion demonstrated the formation of 20α-hydroxy-4-pregnene-3-one and 5α-pregnane-3, 20-dione. The latter compound was further metabolized to 3β-hydroxy-5α-pregnane-20-one, demonstrating that both fetal membranes contain 20α-hydroxysteroid oxidoreductase, 5α-reductase, and 3β-hydroxysteroid oxidoreductase activities [40]. The amnion was found to have relatively higher 5α-reductase activity, while chorion had relatively greater 20α-hydroxysteroid oxidoreductase and 3β-hydroxysteroid oxidoreductase activities [40]. In further studies, it could be demonstrated that the 10–20-fold decrease of 20-hydroxysteroid oxidoreductase activity and the 2–6-fold decrease in 5-reductase activity are observed in human amnion and chorion after 33 weeks of gestation [41]. The type of delivery does not seem to influence these activities [41]. These enzyme activities in amnion and chorion have been partially characterized, including optimal pH, cofactor requirements, Km values, and optimal temperature [274]. The metabolism of C_{21} steroids was also demonstrated using cultured amniotic fluid cells [275]. The data are listed in Table 94.

Considerably more radioactivity (77%–82%) could be extracted from the incubation media than from the tryptinized cell monolayers (7%–10%). The distribution pattern was similar in both. The amount of metabolism increased with time. However, most of the radioactivity was located in the unidentified fractions. The results demonstrate the metabolism of pregnenolone to progesterone, which is further metabolized to 17α-OH and 20α-OH-progesterone. Progesterone is converted to 17α-OH and 20α-OH-progesterone, while 20α-OH-progesterone is changed into progesterone and from there to some extent to 17α-OH-progesterone. These findings indicate that amniotic fluid cells

Table 94. Metabolism of pregnenolone-^{3}H, progesterone-^{3}H and 20α-hydroxyprogesterone-^{3}H in cultures of human amniotic fluid cells [275]

Labeled steroids and incubation	Steroids isolated from the cell monolayers. Percent of ether-extractable radioactivity of isolated steroid				
	Pregnenolone	Progesterone	17α-OH-prog	20α-OH-prog	Unidentified steroid
Pregnenolone-^{3}H					
24 h	61.1%	0.7%	0.3%	0.0%	32.0%
48 h	57.4	1.8	1.1	1.0	31.0
Progesterone-^{3}H					
24 h	–	67.2	0.7	2.1	17.0
48 h	–	62.1	1.3	4.8	16.0
20α-OH-^{3}H					
24 h	–	8.2	1.1	59.2	15.0
48 h	–	16.6	1.9	41.2	11.0
	Steroids isolated from the incubation media from amniotic fluid cell culture. Percent of ether-extractable radioactivity of isolated steroids				
Pregnenolone-^{3}H					
24 h	55.2%	0.8%	0.2%	0.0%	34.0%
48 h	51.7	2.2	0.8	2.0	32.0
Progesterone-^{3}H					
24 h	–	62.2	0.8	1.1	14.0
48 h	–	64.0	1.1	5.2	20.0
20α-OH-Prog-^{3}H					
24 h	–	6.2	0.6	61.2	21.0
48 h	–	15.2	1.2	49.9	14.0

contain 3β-OH-steroid oxidoreductase, 17α-hydroxylase, and 20α-hydroxysteroid oxidoreductase. The enzyme pattern is comparable to the activities described before for amniotic membranes [40].

The metabolism of C_{19} steroids by human fetal membrane or human amniotic epithelium has revealed several enzyme activities. It was demonstrated that steroid sulfatase for the conversion of DS to D is present only in the chorion, located mainly in the microsome fraction [267]. This is in agreement with the findings on estrogen sulfate transfer through the fetal membranes [46, 265]. The free steroid moiety of D is further metabolized to Δ^4-androstenedione, testosterone and 5α-androstane-3,17-dione, reflecting 3β-OH-steroid oxidoreductase, Δ^{5-4}-isomerase activity as well as 5α-reductase activity [267]. 3β-OH-steroid oxidoreductase-Δ^{5-4}-isomerase was also shown by others [42]. The substrate dehydroepiandrosterone-4-^{14}C was converted by human amniotic epithelium from the 7th to the 23rd week of pregnancy into Δ^4-androstenedione, testosterone and Δ^5-androstendiol. Regarding the formation of these metabolites, there was an age dependency. Both enzymes, 3β-OH steroid oxydoreductase and Δ^{5-4}-isomerase activity increased from low values at 7 weeks of gestation to the maximum in the 8th to the 9th weeks followed by a gradual decrease. At 21–23 weeks of gestation these activities are no longer demonstrable. These changes parallel the formation of testosterone by the human fetal testes [276]. Incubating Δ^5-androstenediol-4-^{14}C, the rate of conversion to androstenedione and testosterone was similar [42]. However, formation of 17-oxo- from 17-OH-steroid (conversion of Δ^5-adrostenediol to dehydroepiandrosterone) was significantly elevated in the second trimester [42]. Expanded studies on the metabolism of D and Δ^5-adiol between the 5th and 23rd week of gestation have recently been reported [426] demonstrating a significant increase of steroid hydroxylase and 17β-hydroxysteroid dehydrogenase activity and a decrease of 3β-OH-steroid dehydrogenase/Δ^{5-4}-isomerase activity. Dependence of these steroid metabolizing enzyme activities on fetal sex was not observed [426].

In general, a preponderance of 17-ketone formation from 17,3-hydroxysteroids exists in the human amniotic epithelium [43].

Also, 7α- and 7β-hydroxylase activity of dehydroepiandrosterone was demonstrated in human amniotic epithelium [44]. The 7α-hydroxylase prevailed over 7β-hydroxylation. In incubation studies with chorion, the 7β-epimer was the more abundant metabolite [45]. It was found that 7-hydroxalation progressively increased from fetuses of both sexes from the 7th to the 23rd week of gestation [277]. The activity for 16-hydroxylase was so low in human amniotic epithelium to be neglected from a quantitative point of view [44].

In cultured human amniotic fluid cells testosterone metabolism was proved [278], indicating a metabolic pattern similar to fibroblasts except for lower activity.

Differences in information on 5α-reduced metabolites of testosterone by amniotic fluid cells from a fetus with testicular feminization make the prenatal diagnosis of testicular feminization possible [278]. Furthermore, aromatase activity was demonstrated in the chorion converting Δ^4-androstenedione and D to estrogens [46]. The conversion of E_1 and E_2 is extensive in fetal membranes [46].

These enzyme activities in the human amniotic membranes appear to be subject to regulation by steroids. For membrane sulfatase, it was demonstrated that, for instance, pregnenolone sulfate or cholesterol sulfate are just such competitors [267], and it was found that pregnenolone sulfate and dehydroepiandrosterone sulfate have similar affinities to the enzyme [267]. Therefore, in vivo regulation of steroid metabolism in human amniotic membranes is a complex phenomenon that as yet has not been elucidated.

I. Fate of Steroids Injected into the Amniotic Cavity

The first report on dehydroepiandrosterone injection into the amniotic fluid of a patient with a live anencephalic fetus was made by Frandsen and Stakeman [279]. An increase of urinary estrogen excretion was noticed, particularly in the estrone-estradiol fraction. Similar findings were also obtained in women scheduled for legal abortion [107].

This is most likely due to the use of free D in contrast to the follow-up studies using DS [107]. Such a type of investigation was done by Michie [107] in four pregnancies with live anencephalic fetuses. Estrogen increase in maternal urine and in the amniotic fluid was found. The data are listed in Tables 95 and 96.

Using DS, mainly an increase of estriol in maternal urine as well as in amniotic fluid was found [107]. Later in normal and other abnormal pregnancies, intra-amniotic injection of DS was done [280–282]. With intra-amniotic injection of 200 μg DS, Hausknecht and Mandelbaum [280] obtained the data listed in Table 97.

A rise of urinary estriol is clearly demonstrated in case I where the infant had been dead in utero. The diminished and shorter rise of estriol is most likely due to direct transfer of DS from the amniotic cavity via the amniotic membranes and the placenta. This is supported by the findings that intra-amniotic instillation of 250 mg DS did not change the rate of maternal estriol and estrone excretion with sulfatase deficiency [281]. In an extensive clinical study, 12 normal pregnant women and 33 cases with abnormal pregnancies were examined [282]. In the normal cases, the total urinary estrogen excretion

Table 95. Effect of intra-amniotic injection of 250 mg of sodium dehydroepiandrosterone sulfate on urinary estrogen excretion in four women with a live anencephalic fetus [107]

		Urine concentration (μg/24 h)				
		Estriol	Estradiol	Estrone	Total estrogens	Estriol/ estrone and estradiol
Case No. 1	Before DS	433	60	30	523	4.8
	After DS	1028	144	39	1211	5.6
2	Before DS	995	61	24	1080	11.7
	After DS	2017	94	57	2168	13.4
3	Before DS	2219	195	87	2501	7.8
	After DS	3333	146	73	3260	14.0
4	Before DS	3185	130	100	3435	12.7
	After DS	5080	256	119	5455	13.5

Table 96. Effect of intra-amniotic injection of 250 mg of sodium dehydroepiandrosterone sulfate on amniotic fluid estrogen levels in four women with a live anencephalic fetus [107]

		Amniotic fluid concentration (μg/100 ml)		
		Estriol	Estradiol	Estrone
Case No. 1	Before DS	1.5	0.1	0.5
	24 h after DS	1.7	0.1	0.2
2	Before DS	0.8	0.2	0.2
	24 h after DS	1.1	0.2	–
3	Before DS	5.3	0.2	0.3
	24 h after DS	8.8	0.3	0.2
4	Before DS	4.2	–	–
	24 h after DS	8.6	0.3	–
Mean	Before DS	2.95	0.13	0.25
	24 h after DS	5.05	0.23	0.10

Table 97. Maternal urinary estriol excretion after intra-amniotic injection of 200 mg DS in normal and abnormal gestation [280]

	Estriol (mg/24 h)			
	Preinjection time	24 h after injection	48 h after injection	72 h after injection
Normal gestation				
Case No. 1	27.3	38.6 (+41%)	42.4	28.6
2	24.8	40.4 (+62%)	36.4	25.1
3	19.9	33.7 (+69%)	29.7	21.6
4	34.9	51.9 (+48%)	41.5	–
Abnormal gestation				
Case No. I	1.9	2.3 (+21%)	1.9	0.9
II	4.2	8.9 (+111%)	10.8	6.5
III	9.9	15.2 (+52%)	15.8	10.1

exceeded at least more than 100% with an average of 147.6% ± 46.6 (SD). In 28 of 33 pathologic pregnancies, the increment did not reach 100%. An average increment of 48.6% ± 19.2 (SD) was found [282]. It is noteworthy that in 24 pathologic cases with borderline to normal urinary estriol excretion, the increment after DS injection did not reach 100%, while in two cases with anencephaly, in one case with mongolism, and in one case with congenital nanism with low urinary estriol excretion the increment always exceeded 100% [282].

Intra-amniotic DS injection not only changes maternal estrogen excretion or amniotic fluid estrogen concentration [107, 279–282], but also alters C_{19} steroid levels [283]. It was found that 180 min after DS injection, the peak concentration of the C_{18} steroids appeared except for estrone, which reached its maximum at 120 min [283]. For the C_{19} steroids, the same temporal relationship was found. Seventy-five percent of the incremental estrogens were 16-hydroxylated, and among the C_{19} steroid fractions 16α-OH-D was isolated with the highest concentration. The values for Δ^4-androstenedione and testosterone were almost equal. Already 15 min after intra-amniotic injection, a significant quantity of radiolabeled metabolites appeared in the maternal circulation and increased up to 3 h. Since 75% of all recovered metabolites were 16-hydroxylated, about 25% do not seem to pass the fetal liver and consequently reach the placenta without 16α-hydroxylation. Since small amounts of unmetabolized labeled D were found in the maternal circulation, passage through the amniotic membranes is likely [283].

A comparison of intra-amniotic (100–200 mg) and intravenous (100 mg) administration of DS was done measuring unconjugated E_2, T, and total E_3 in 26 women with midtrimester abortion. E_3 and T levels in amniotic fluid rose significantly ($P < 0.01$) 1–6 h after the intra-amniotic injection, while the E_3 level remained unchanged. Similar changes in the maternal circulation were seen for E_2 and T but also for E_3. However, after the intravenous injection of DS, E_3 remained unchanged in the maternal circulation. This indicates that the intra-amniotically injected DS is taken up by the fetus, for instance, by fetal swallowing [284].

Intra-amniotic injection of labeled E_2 and E_3 resulted in formation of E_4, a metabolite exclusively formed in the fetus [285, 286]. These results are in agreement with data obtained by direct injection of labeled E_2 into the peritoneal cavity of the fetus [285]. The influence of steroid conjugation on the fate of intra-amniotically injected estrogens has already been detailed [264–266, 268]. Injection of E_3 sulfate into the amniotic fluid resulted in a peak excretion of estriol in the maternal urine 4–8 h and after 36 h an average of 35.7% of the administered sulfate had been excreted [287]. Attempts to use the procedure as a placental function test failed since the recovery of E_3 in maternal urine was similar in normal and abnormal pregnancies [288].

Studies on the effect of intra-amniotically injected estriol sulfate revealed marginal improvement of the response of the uterus to intra-amniotically saline-induced abortions [289], but in postmaturity no difference to a placebo group could be noticed [290].

Interesting findings have emerged after intra-amniotic injection of cortisol [291, 292]. A dose of 500 mg of cortisol caused a decrease of estriol in amniotic fluid after 48 h from 82.5 μg/100 ml to 47.4 mg/100 ml, an increase of cortisol from 5.5 mg/100 ml to 41.9 mg/100 ml, and an increase of progesterone from 22.6 ng/ml to 61.9 ng/ml. The amniotic fluid parameters for fetal lung maturity improved [286]. In the venous cord blood, estriol was depressed (17.2 versus 79.0 μg/100 ml in a normal control group). The cortisol level was increased (21.3 versus 18.7 μg/100 ml), and marked elevation of progesterone was found (497.6 versus 109.1 ng/ml).

In maternal blood, estriol concentration decreased, cortisol levels were elevated, but progesterone values remained essentially unchanged [291]. A similar study [292] confirmed these findings in maternal blood for E_3 and also demonstrated a decrease in estriol, while a nonsignificantly raised progesterone concentration was found. Spontaneous onset of labor was noted in the face of the decreasing estrogen levels and dominance of progesterone. Induction of labor by such procedure was demonstrated in comparison to a control group, and a significant difference ($P < 0.001$) was found [293].

J. Binding of Steroids in Human Amniotic Fluid

Proteins for binding, such as albumin, testosterone-estradiol-binding globulin (TEBG), and corticosteroid-binding globulin (CBG) are present in amniotic fluid [294]. The results of the measurements of the free fractions of the steroids were obtained by equilibrium dialysis, and the specific protein-bound fraction was calculated by the specific displacement with the charcoal absorption technique in pregnancies at 14–18 weeks of gestation [294]. The results are listed in Table 98.

Table 98. Steroid concentration and the percent of free and specific protein-bound fraction of steroids in amniotic fluid 14–18 weeks of gestation [294]

Steroid	n	Fetal sex	Concentration (pg/ml; mean ± SEM)	Fraction (%; mean ± SEM)			
				Free	n	Specific protein-bound	n
Estrone	67	Male	256 ± 18	28.5 ± 1.4	10	1.5 ± 0.5	10
	29	Female	303 ± 30	25.0 ± 2.2	10	2.1 ± 0.6	10
Estradiol	67	Male	85 ± 5.7	15.6 ± 0.6	66	11.1 ± 0.7	61
	30	Female	102 ± 15.0	14.5 ± 0.8	30	14.6 ± 1.0	26
Androstene-dione	63	Male	658 ± 33.0	32.3 ± 2.7	10	1.9 ± 0.3	10
	29	Female	360 ± 28.0	27.1 ± 2.7	10	3.6 ± 0.7	10
Testosterone	63	Male	277 ± 16.0	13.6 ± 0.6	66	28.5 ± 1.0	60
	29	Female	41 ± 3.7	11.7 ± 0.7	30	34.7 ± 1.3	26
Progesterone	67	Male	55000 ± 3400	20.6 ± 1.2	10	3.3 ± 0.6	10
	30	Female	54000 ± 4500	20.0 ± 1.6	10	5.8 ± 1.0	10

There are significant high-affinity protein-bound fractions for E_2 and T and only minimal for E_1, androstenedione, and progesterone. Furthermore, a small but significant sex difference in the specific protein-bound fraction of E_2, progesterone and the free fraction of T was measured [294]. In general, the free fractions of all the steroids examined were higher in the amniotic fluid than in the maternal plasma, but the reverse was true for the specific protein-bound fractions [294]. The much higher free fraction of the steroids in amniotic fluid is explained by the low protein concentration amniotic fluid [295]. As pregnancy advances, the protein concentration in amniotic fluid decreases [295] and, therefore, with an increase in steroid production the biologically active fraction of steroids in amniotic fluid can increase continuously.

For cortisol a high-affinity binding protein in amniotic fluid was established [296]. This protein resembles corticosteroid-binding globulin (CBG) characterized by heat stability up to 50 °C and failure to precipitate by 50% ammonium sulfate treatment [296]. There are distinct differences to testosterone-estradiol-binding globulin (TEGB), also established in amniotic fluid [297].

Throughout pregnancy, the association constant and the binding capacity of cortisol do not change significantly in normal and abnormal gestation as listed in Table 99 [296].

Table 99. Association constants and binding capacity of cortisol binding in human amniotic fluid (mean ± SEM) [246]

Type of pregnancy	n	Ka × $10^8 M^{-1}$	Binding capacity (ng/100 ml)
14–20 weeks	7	3.90 ± 1.25	860 ± 269
Term	10	3.86 ± 0.42	577 ± 138
Anencephaly (17–18 weeks)	2	3.03 ± 0.31	878 ± 109

Since cortisol increases in amniotic fluid throughout pregnancy [71, 144, 150, 158, 161, 162, 172, 253], unchanged cortisol binding capacity of amniotic fluid results in an increase in the concentration of unbound cortisol in amniotic fluid toward the end of pregnancy. The biologic significance of this is not known at present.

Besides the specific steroid-binding globulins, there is also binding of steroids to albumin. The binding is more extensive to human albumin than to cow albumin. This was first demonstrated for D [298] and confirmed for E_3 and E_1 [188]. Furthermore, it was demonstrated that E_3 was less bound than E_1, independent from the albumin concentration, and that binding increased with albumin concentration (Fig. 15 [188]).

That indeed 16-hydroxylated steroids are less bound than the corresponding non-16-hydroxylated precursors was demonstrated with three steroid pairs [188]. The data are listed in Table 100.

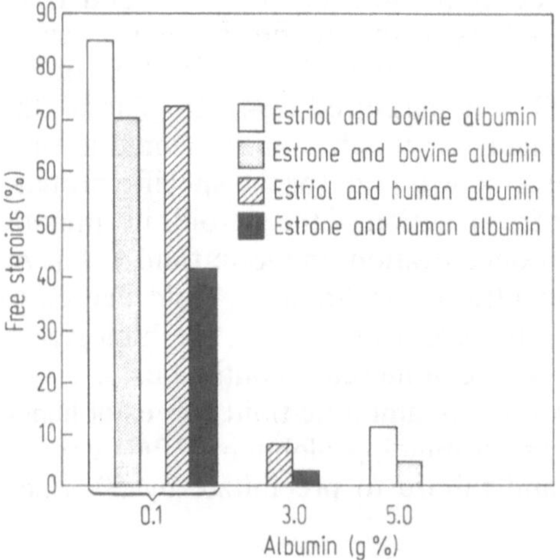

Fig. 15. E_1 and E_3 binding to human and bovine albumin. (Schindler 1972 [188])

These results support the conclusions that differences in nonspecific binding contribute to the excretion and regulation of steroids in amniotic fluid. Smith et al. [299] consider even the large number of correlations between estriol concentration in various compartments as evidence for the low affinity of estriol for binding proteins as compared to the non-16-hydroxylated steroids.

Table 100. Percent free steroid at various albumin concentrations [188]

Steroid	Albumin concentration (g%)		
	0.1	1.0	3.0
Estriol	72.1	23.3	7.3
Estrone	41.6	10.5	2.1
16α-OH-D	72.8	14.8	5.0
D	36.8	6.5	2.8
16-OH-preg	56.7	14.0	5.8
Preg	21.7	4.1	2.2

K. Proteohormones in Human Amniotic Fluid

I. Luteinizing Hormone (LH)

The replacement of biologic methods by specific radioimmunoassays has also increased the possibilities for studying protein hormones in human amniotic fluid. However, until recently it was not possible to differentiate by RIA between LH and human chorionic gonadotropin (HCG). After the detection of structure differences in the β-subunit between LH and HCG [300], the development of antisera against the respective β-units was possible. Radioimmunoassay with such antisera yielded measurable levels of LH in amniotic fluid that were compared to fetal serum, fetal pituitary content, and pituitary excretion of LH [301]. The results are shown in Table 101.

Prior to 12 weeks of gestation, LH in amniotic fluid is low or absent. Between 12–20 weeks of gestation, a rise of LH concentration is evident with significant sex difference ($P < 0.001$) of LH in amniotic fluid as well as in

Table 101. LH in human amniotic fluid, fetal serum, and fetal pituitary gland [301]

Fetal age	Fetal sex	LH (ng pure LH; mean ± SEM)							
		Amniotic fluid	n	Fetal serum	n	Pituitary content	n	Pituitary concentration	n
<12 weeks	Male	1.0 ± 0.2	15	–	–	6.4 ± 2.3	4	4.5 ± 1.9	4
	Female	1.4 ± 0.3	7	0.6	1	4.1	1	2.9	1
10–20 weeks	Male	3.5 ± 0.5	41	5.1 ± 0.8	17	73.4 ± 12.9	18	15.2 ± 2.3	18
	Female	10.8 ± 1.1	31	14.5 ± 3.1	9	342.0 ± 118.0	13	53.6 ± 9.1	13
32 weeks – term	Male	0.6 ± 0.08	7	–	–	–	–	–	–
	Female	0.4 ± 0.042	20	–	–	–	–	–	–

Table 102. LH in human amniotic fluid according to the fetal sex [302]

Weeks of gestation	Fetal sex	LH (ng pure LH; mean ± SEM)	n	P[a]
16	Male	11.5 ± 0.6	20	<0.01
	Female	18.9 ± 0.9	20	
18	Male	15.3 ± 1.4	12	$0.05 < P < 0.1$
	Female	20.4 ± 2.4	10	
20	Male	13.7 ± 0.7	17	$0.001 < P < 0.01$
	Female	18.5 ± 1.1	19	

[a] P, Significance of sex differences

fetal serum and pituitary tissue. Confirmatory data were recently published as listed in Table 102 [302].

These peculiarities of LH concentration are most likely due to sex differences in steroid concentration, as mentioned in previous chapters, as well as by feedback regulation. The high levels of LH in the female fetuses appear to correlate with fetal ovarian development [303] and 3-β-hydroxysteroid dehydrogenase activity of the interstitial cells of the fetal ovary and in vitro metabolic activity of the fetal ovary [304], indicating that gonadal development is connected with fetal LH secretion and reflected in LH activity in amniotic fluid.

II. Follicle-Stimulating Hormone (FSH)

Several studies on FSH levels in amniotic fluid are available [86, 94, 95, 210, 210a, 301]. Similar to LH, there is a significant sex difference at midgestation. The data are summarized in Table 103. These data demonstrate a significant sex difference between 12 and 20 weeks of gestation. In one study, it could be shown that up to 13 weeks of gestation no sex differences exist for FSH in human amniotic fluid [210a]. In another investigation, differences were absent below 12 weeks of gestation [301]. A comparison of FSH in amniotic fluid, fetal serum, and fetal pituitary gland is shown in Table 104.

As shown by Clements et al. [301], there is a significant correlation between the FSH concentration in amniotic fluid versus fetal serum ($P<0.001$) and amniotic fluid versus pituitary concentration ($P<0.001$). This indicates that the FSH content of amniotic fluid reflects fetal pituitary activity [204]. These

Table 103. FSH in human amniotic fluid

Weeks of gestation	n	Fetal sex	FSH (mIU)		FSH (ng/ml; mean ± SEM)	P[a]	Ref.
			Mean	Range			
14–20	60	Male	0.7	0.5– 8.6	–	<0.01	94
	36	Female	7.5	2.0– 32.0	–		
15–26	11	Male	2.3	0.6– 4.0	–	<0.01	95
	9	Female	20.4	1.6– 50.0	–		
12–20	41	Male	–	–	0.1 ± 0.02	<0.001	301
	31	Female	–	–	0.6 ± 0.1		
32–term	5	Male	–	–	0.3 ± 0.08	NS	301
	19	Female	–	–	0.2 ± 0.01		
14–22	66	Male	1.3	–	–	<0.01	46
	33	Female	10.1	–	–		
16–20	166	Male	8.5	6.3– 10.9	–	–	210
	187	Female	18.4	7.6– 93.4	–		
14–22	35	Male	6.8	5.0– 23.0	–	<0.001	210a
	41	Female	37.7	5.0–150	–		

[a] P, Significance of sex differences

Table 104. FSH in human amniotic fluid, fetal serum, and fetal pituitary gland [301]

Fetal age	Fetal sex	FSH (ng pure FSH; mean ± SEM)							
		Amniotic fluid	n	Fetal serum	n	Pituitary content	n	Pituitary concentration	n
<12 weeks	Male	<0.1	15	0.1 ± 0.02	3	0.4 ± 0.06	4	0.2 ± 0.04	4
	Female	<0.1	7	0.8	2	0.5	1	0.4	1
12–20 weeks	Male	0.1 ± 0.02	41	0.3 ± 0.04	29	1.4 ± 0.2	18	0.3 ± 0.03	18
	Female	0.6 ± 0.1	31	5.4 ± 1.4	15	42.8 ± 19.0	13	5.3 ± 1.7	13
32 weeks –term	Male	0.3 ± 0.08	5	0.1 ± 0.4	4	–	–	–	–
	Female	0.2 ± 0.01	19	<0.1 ± 0.4	29	–	–	–	–

differences in FSH concentration are most likely determined by differences in fetal gonadal steroid secretion. There is a high testosterone level in the male fetus at 10–20 weeks of gestation [305], leading to feedback inhibition of gonadotropin secretion in the male at that time, but most likely not via estradiol, which is present at midgestation in both female and male fetuses. The absence of FSH suppression in the midgestation fetus indicates that hypothalamic and/or pituitary estrogen feedback is not operating at that time. The subsequent decline of FSH to low levels at term could reflect feedback maturation [301]. FSH measurements in combination with testosterone concentrations in amniotic fluid might indicate laboratory error in prenatal caryotype diagnosis [306].

In one study, it could be shown that up to 13 weeks of gestation no sex differences exist for FSH in human amniotic fluid [210a]. In another investigation, differences were absent below 12 weeks of gestation [301].

The predictability of fetal sex by quantitation of FSH in amniotic fluid was reported to be between 45% [210] and 95% [86]. An improvement was achieved up to 100% by simultaneous measurement of FSH and T [86, 94, 210]. The T/FSH ratio was also used [92, 210], and improvement of fetal sex assessment was found [210]. The levels of T and FSH in amniotic fluid are inversely proportionate [210].

III. Human Chorionic Gonadotropin (HCG)

Gonadotropic activity in human amniotic fluid was first reported by Brunner [307]. Development of specific radioimmunoassays have enabled the quantitation of HCG in amniotic fluid in normal and abnormal conditions. The patterns of HCG in amniotic fluid parallels those in fetal and maternal blood and urine [301, 308] with a maximum concentration 12–13 weeks of gestation [301, 306]. Data on normal amniotic fluid are compiled in Table 105.

There are discrepancies in the results regarding fetal sex differences of HCG in amniotic fluid as listed in Table 103. In maternal plasma, such differences have been reported by a number of investigators [309–313]. The relationship of HCG concentration in maternal blood and amniotic fluid and cord blood is shown in Table 106.

Table 105. HCG in human amniotic fluid (mean ± SEM)

Weeks of gestation	n	Type of method, type of standard	Fetal sex	HCG	P[a]	Ref.
<12	17	β-HCG-RIA (ng/ml)	Male	933 ± 193	NS	301
	6	1 ng = 5 mIU 2ndIS	Female	1139 ± 407		
12–20	42	1 ng = 5 mIU 2ndIS	Male	589 ± 64	NS	
	31	1 ng = 5 mIU 2ndIS	Female	789 ± 86		
32–term	7	1 ng = 5 mIU 2ndIS	Male	42 ± 13	NS	
	20	1 ng = 5 mIU 2ndIS	Female	57 ± 8		
11	1	HCG-RIA (IU/ml)	–	100	–	316
20–28	7		–	1.94	–	
32–41	13		–	1.99	–	
42–43	7		–	1.41	–	
16	23	HCG-RIA (IU/ml)	Male	5.2 ± 1.0	NS	302
	20		Female	4.1 ± 0.8		
18	12		Male	3.8 ± 0.8	NS	
	10		Female	3.0 ± 0.6		
20	17		Male	2.2 ± 0.4	NS	
	19		Female	2.6 ± 0.4		
12–20	60	HCG-RIA (ng LER 907/ml)	Male	14.6 ± 1.1	<0.025	208
	39		Female	19.7 ± 1.6		
17–20	10	HCG hemagglutination reaction (IU/ml)	Male and female	< 1.25 – 5.0	–	314
Term	18	HCG hemagglutination reaction (IU/ml)	Male and female	0.7 ± 0.1	–	315
Term	23	HCG biologic method (IU/ml)	Male and female	0.75 ± 0.3	–	306
Term	–	HCG-RIA (IU/ml)	Male	0.49 ± 0.08	–	309
			Female	0.30 ± 0.05		
	62		Male and female	0.38 ± 0.04		
Term	6	HCG-RIA (IU/ml)	Male and female	0.72 ± 0.25	–	310
33–35	10	β-HCG-RIA (ng/ml)	Male and female	132.3	–	131

[a] P, Significance of sex differences

In maternal blood, significantly higher concentrations of HCG are present and in amniotic fluid higher levels than in cord blood (Table 106). A highly significant correlation ($P < 0.001$) was found for HCG in maternal serum and amniotic fluid [302], while others reported a highly significant correlation ($P < 0.001$) between amniotic fluid and cord blood [301]. Again others were unable to establish such correlations [314]. Maternal dexamethasone treatment

Table 106. HCG in maternal blood, amniotic fluid and cord blood

Weeks of gestation	HCG (mean ± SEM)				Type of standard	Ref.
	Fetal sex	Maternal blood	Amniotic fluid	Cord blood		
38–42	Male/female	9.45 ± 0.93	0.38 ± 0.04	0.02 ± 0.003	IU/ml	309
	Male	6.44 ± 0.82	0.49 ± 0.08	0.02 ± 0.004	IU/ml	
	Female	13.62 ± 1.62	0.30 ± 0.05	0.02 ± 0.004	IU/ml	
12	Male	–	933 ± 193	283 ± 140	ng/ml	301
	Female	–	1139 ± 407	213 ± 93	ng/ml	
12–20	Male	–	589 ± 64	69 ± 13	ng/ml	
	Female	–	783 ± 86	107 ± 20	ng/ml	
16	Male	9.23 ± 0.6	5.22 ± 1.04	–	IU/ml	302
	Female	9.43 ± 0.5	4.16 ± 0.81	–	IU/ml	
18	Male	7.49 ± 0.5	3.86 ± 0.89	–	IU/ml	
	Female	8.24 ± 0.5	3.01 ± 0.64	–	IU/ml	
20	Male	4.22 ± 0.4	2.26 ± 0.48	–	IU/ml	
	Female	4.64 ± 0.3	2.69 ± 0.48	–	IU/ml	
Term	Male/female	48.3 ± 22.6	0.72 ± 0.25	0.12 ± 0.01	IU/ml	310

for fetal lung maturation had no influence on amniotic fluid and blood HCG levels [131].

Only few data are available on pathologic conditions of pregnancy. Early studies on Rh incompatibility did not find elevated HCG levels in amniotic fluid although raised concentrations were determined in maternal blood [315].

In 16 Rh-sensitized women, HCG in amniotic fluid was 0.40 ± 0.08 IU/ml while in normal cases a level of 0.73 ± 0.18 IU/ml was present [315]. Later on, significantly elevated levels of HCG were measured in amniotic fluid in Rh incompatibility [306, 308], depending on the severity of sensitization. While in pregnancy grouped in Liley zone I and II the level of HCG was similar to normal, a comparison of patients from zone I and II with zone III revealed a significant difference ($P < 0.001$). The data are listed in Table 107. In the last study [308], maternal blood HCG was also raised according to the severity of Rh incompatibility.

Table 107. HCG in amniotic fluid of normal pregnancies and in pregnancies with Rh incompatibility

	n	HCG (IU/ml)	Ref.
Rh incompatibility			
Liley zone I and II	36	0.58	306
	41	0.45	308, 309
Liley zone III	10	1.5	306
	11	15.6	308, 309
Control group	18	0.75	306
	62	0.38	308, 309

Significantly elevated levels were also found in diabetes [306]. In ten cases, the mean HCG concentration in amniotic fluid was 1.81 IU/ml, while in the control group 0.61 IU/ml were found [306]. This reflects the increased HCG production of the placenta in these conditions [311].

IV. Human Placental Lactogen (HPL)

The presence of this protein hormone in amniotic fluid was first described in 1965 [312, 313, 317]. Numerous investigations have been done in the mean time. Results on HPL in amniotic fluid in normal and complicated pregnancies are listed in Table 108.

Table 108. HPL in human amniotic fluid

Weeks of gestation	n	Clinical diagnosis	HPL (μg/ml)	Ref.
11	1	Normal	0.013	316
20–28	7	Normal	0.117	
32–41	13	Normal	0.198	
42–43	7	Normal	0.154	
36–41	–	Normal	0.550	318
20	10	Normal	0.150	319
Term	7	Normal	0.500	
Term	–	Normal	0.547	309
38–42	51	Normal	0.610	320
11–13	10	Normal	0.414	321
14–15	9	Normal	0.458	
16–19	9	Normal	0.448	
20–23	6	Normal	0.302	
24–27	4	Normal	0.573	
28–31	5	Normal	0.695	
32–35	9	Normal	0.686	
36–40	8	Normal	0.443	
24–27	10	Normal	0.616	322
28–31	14	Normal	0.603	
32–35	19	Normal	0.671	
24–27	12	Severe Rh in-	0.826	322
28–31	13	compatibility	0.721	
32–35	18	Liley zone III	0.982	
32	2	Rh incompatibility	0.178	323
33–36	3	without exchange	0.501	
37–40	4	transfer	0.607	
32	6		0.696	
33–36	12		0.500	
37–40	7		0.476	
32	3	Rh incompatibility with hydrops	0.533	
33–36	2	fetalis or fetal	0.450	
37–40	1	death	0.530	
Term	–	Normal	0.430	310
29–34	16	Normal	0.600	324
35–40	10	Normal	0.770	

Continued next page

Table 108 (continued)

Weeks of gestation	n	Clinical diagnosis	HPL (μg/ml)	Ref.
14–23	7	Normal	0.475	325
28–30	11	Normal	0.59	326
31–33	13	Normal	0.65	
34–36	19	Normal	0.85	
37–39	31	Normal	0.80	
40–42	76	Normal	0.65	
43	35	Prolonged	0.48	
28–33	18	Normal	0.78	327
34–36	19	Normal	0.85	
37–39	45	Normal	0.72	
40–42	80	Normal	0.64	
28–33	15	Gestosis	0.50	
34–36	12	Gestosis	0.59	
37–39	10	Gestosis	0.41	
40–42	6	Gestosis	0.17	
37–39	30	Normal	0.8	328
37–39	16	Diabetes class A	1.2	

Table 109. HPL in maternal serum and amniotic fluid

Weeks of gestation	HPL (μg/ml)				Ref.
	Maternal serum	n	Amniotic fluid	n	
20	1.8	12	0.150	10	319
Term	5.5	30	0.500	10	
Term	6.34	–	0.547	–	309
Term	7.7	–	0.43	–	310
36–41	5.4	–	0.55	–	318
38–42	7.94	51	0.61	51	320
11–13	0.40	10	0.41	16	321
14–15	0.88	9	0.45	9	
16–19	1.70	9	0.44	9	
20–23	1.72	6	0.30	6	
24–27	2.76	4	0.57	4	
18–31	4.12	5	0.69	5	
32–35	5.45	9	0.68	9	
36–40	10.23	8	0.44	8	
28–30	3.05		0.59		326
31–33	4.38		0.65		
34–36	6.70		0.85		
37–39	6.20		0.80		
40–42	5.37		0.65		
43+	2.75		0.48		

In normal amniotic fluid, there is an increase of HPL during gestation, but the pattern is not unique [316, 319, 321, 326]. The highest values have been found around 34–36 weeks of gestation [321, 326, 327]. Thereafter, a decrease occurs [321, 326, 327] and is most obvious in prolonged pregnancy [316, 326].

It appears that there is no correlation between amniotic fluid volume and HPL concentration in normal amniotic fluid [321] and in amniotic fluid from pregnancies with Rh incompatibility [329].

According to experimental studies [330], it was clearly demonstrated that radioactively labeled HPL may pass from the maternal to the liquor side of isolated chorion and amnion or in a reverse direction by diffusion. There is indeed a considerable concentration gradient from the maternal circulation to amniotic fluid. The level in amniotic fluid is below one eighth that found in maternal serum during the last trimester [309, 310, 319, 321, 326, 331, 332]. Available data are listed in Table 109.

There is a decreasing HPL ratio in maternal serum and amniotic fluid from 1.1 to 0.04 during the last 5 weeks of pregnancy; the difference was statistically significant [321]. This could either reflect decreasing transfer through the amnion and chorion or increasing metabolism of HPL in amniotic fluid [321]. Very little HPL is found in the fetal circulation [309, 310, 332], and there is no significant difference of HPL concentration in the umbilical artery and umbilical vein [316].

Comparisons of HPL levels in cord blood and amniotic fluid are summarized in Table 110.

Table 110. HPL in cord blood and amniotic fluid

Weeks of gestation	HPL (μg/ml)				Ref.
	Cord blood	n	Amniotic fluid	n	
Last trimester	0.010[a]	29	–		316
	0.014[b]	32			
32–41	–	–	0.198	13	
Term	0.027	–	0.547	–	309
Term	0.022	72	0.43	72	310
Term	0.045	55	0.76	8	332

[a] Arterial cord blood
[b] Venous cord blood

There is an over tenfold difference between HPL concentration in amniotic fluid and cord blood and a 100–400-fold difference between HPL levels in maternal blood and cord blood. Data on correlations of HPL levels in the various compartments have been obtained. A significant correlation ($P < 0.01$) of HPL values with gestational age in normal pregnancy has been found, but not in preeclampsia and Rh incompatibility [324].

By comparing HPL in amniotic fluid and placental weight, some authors found significant correlations [328, 329] while others did not [320, 324]. Similar discrepancies were found when correlations between HPL in amniotic fluid and infant weight were sought [324, 328]. Several studies have indicated parallelism [318] and significant correlations ($P < 0.005 - P < 0.001$) between maternal blood and HPL in amniotic fluid [309, 320, 322, 333], but this could not be confirmed in other investigations on normal as well as pathologic pregnancies. No correlation existed between HPL levels in amniotic fluid and cord blood [309].

Studies on fetal lung maturation have shown that with an increasing L/S ratio, there is a decrease in HPL concentration in amniotic fluid [334], which reflects the decrease of HPL in amniotic fluid toward term as previously described.

In pathologic conditions of pregnancy, most studies were done on Rh incompatibility [308, 318, 322–324, 329, 331, 335–337]. Some of the reports have found elevated levels, particularly when the severity of the condition was taken into account. In mild and moderately affected cases, no major changes compared to normals were seen. Some of the data are listed in Table 111.

Table 111. HPL in human amniotic fluid in Rh incompatibility

Weeks of gestation	HPL (μg/liter)						Ref.
	Normal pregnancy	n	Mild to moderate Rh incompatibility	n	Severe Rh incompatibility	n	
24–27	0.61	10	–	–	0.82	12	322
28–31	0.60	14	–	–	0.72	13	
32–35	0.67	19			0.98	18	
–	–	–	0.62	41	1.96	11	308

The levels in amniotic fluid parallel the changes in maternal serum [308, 318] and were significantly ($P<0.001$) correlated [329]. Intrauterine transfusions can result in normalization of the HPL concentration in amniotic fluid [323].

It was concluded from one study [329] that levels above 1 μg/ml at any stage of pregnancy suggest an unfavorable outcome for the fetus, while levels less than 0.7 μg/ml after the 28th week of gestation indicated a favorable outcome. The earliest rise was noted in the most severe cases. After the 28th week of gestation, there was a significant difference ($P<0.001$) between those pregnancies in which the babies survived and those in which they did not [329]. A correlation of fetal condition in Rh incompatibility with the maternal serum/amniotic fluid ratio for HPL was found in 74% [331]. High

Table 112. HPL in human amniotic fluid in pregnancies complicated by diabetes

Weeks of gestation	HPL (μg/ml)			Ref.
	Normal pregnancy	Gestational diabetes	Juvenile diabetes	
33–36	0.79	0.82	0.93	323
37–39	0.80	1.2	–	328

ratios in Rh incompatibility have been measured and appeared to be clinically useful [338]. In contrast to most investigations, lack of correlation between the level of HPL in amniotic fluid and the severity of Rh incompatibility was stated by Ylikorkala and Tuimala [324].

Three studies reported on the level of HPL in amniotic fluid and diabetes [323, 324, 328]. In two studies, elevated concentrations were measured [323, 328] as summarized in Table 112.

Two studies give data on HPL in amniotic fluid in pregnancies complicated by preeclampsia [324, 328], while one study could not detect differences in concentration compared to normal values [324]. Another study [328] found significantly lower values, as listed in Table 113.

Table 113. HPL in human amniotic fluid in pregnancies complicated by preeclampsia [328]

Weeks of gestation	HPL (μg/ml; mean ± SEM)				P[a]
	Normal pregnancy	n	Gestosis	n	
28–33	0.78 ± 0.10	18	0.50 ± 0.004	15	<0.01
34–36	0.85 ± 0.08	19	0.59 ± 0.05	12	<0.01
37–39	0.72 ± 0.05	45	0.41 ± 0.07	10	<0.001
40–42	0.64 ± 0.002	80	0.17 ± 0.06	6	<0.001

[a] P, Significance between normal and abnormal conditions

In pregnant patients with hypertension or renal disease, the HPL values in amniotic fluid were in the same range as in normal pregnancy [323]. A wide range of values (0.036–2.0 μg/ml) were found in six cases with hydramnios [323].

In a number of pathologic conditions, such as placental insufficiency, diabetes mellitus, intrauterine trauma, and Rh incompatibility, a high maternal serum/amniotic fluid HPL ratio was found [338]. It was concluded that a quotient below 10% indicated a birth weight above the 25th percentile and a healthy newborn. Values above 20% were associated with intrauterine fetal death. The clinical usefulness of such a procedure was pointed out [338].

V. Prolactin (Prl)

Measurements of Prl by radioimmunoassay have been available since 1971 when Prl concentrations in amniotic fluid were first reported [339]. It was realized that the level of Prl is far greater in amniotic fluid than in maternal and fetal blood [319]. These findings by radioimmunoassay were confirmed by bioassay indicating that Prl in amniotic fluid exists as molecules with both immunologic and biologic activity [340]. The existence of Prl in small amounts (0.01 IU/ml) has already been measured by bioassay [341].

A number of studies have been done for the isolation and characterization of Prl in amniotic fluid [341a]. Prl from amniotic fluid and plasma was found to be a single biologically and immunologically active protein hormone distinct from human growth hormone (HGH) on the basis of its free mobility and net charge. The molecular size was not significantly different from that of HGH [342]. Later on, a mixture of Prl isohormones with high immunologic and biologic activity was isolated and characterized [343]. More detailed studies on "small" and "big" isohormones in human amniotic fluid have followed [344, 345]; other investigations have also reported on isolation and characterization of Prl in this biologic fluid [346].

There is a lack of correlation between Prl levels in amniotic fluid and maternal as well as cord blood [347, 348]; bromocryptine therapy suppressed maternal Prl but not Prl levels in amniotic fluid [349]. Differences in the percentage of "small" and "big" Prl were also found. The size heterogeneity of Prl in amniotic fluid differed from maternal Prl to a greater degree than it did from fetal Prl [277]. Since considerable amounts of Prl in amniotic fluid are found during the first trimester [350], the fetal pituitary does not appear to be the major source even though fetal pituitary Prl is present in early pregnancy [350]. In pregnant rhesus monkeys, neither maternal hypophysectomy nor fetal death decreased the Prl concentration in amniotic fluid [49]. Therefore, beside maternal or fetal pituitary, a different source of prolactin in amniotic fluid had to be present. Indeed, in a study investigating amnion, chorion, placenta, and decidual tissue taken from term pregnancy, the decidua alone contained significant quantities of Prl [48]. The amount of Prl released far exceeded the decrease in tissue content during incubation. Therefore, the decidua was considered by these investigators to be a major source of Prl in amniotic fluid since sufficient Prl was present in the decidua to account for the amount found in the amniotic fluid [48]. Other investigators could not seperate chorion and decidual tissue sufficiently and studied both tissues together [50, 51]. Golander et al. [50] found that explants of the chorion-decidua secreted Prl over the entire 6-day culture period at a relatively constant rate with a daily secretion of 294 ± 34 ng/10 mg wet weight of tissue. Similar to the previous study [48], the total amount of Prl released over the 6-day period exceeded by far (1,800%) the amount in the tissue before culture. The amnion or placenta released less than 10 ng Prl during the first 24 h of incubation and none thereafter [50]. A similar study [51] revealed prior to incubation a significantly higher Prl concentration ($P < 0.005$) in the decidua-chorion (27.7 ± 5.7 ng/mg protein) and amnion (19.07 ± 6.9 ng/mg protein) than in the placenta (3.1 ± 0.5 ng/mg protein). After incubation, the decidua-chorion released significantly more Prl into the culture medium than did the amnion and placenta. After 72 h of culture, the Prl concentration of the decidua-chorion remained high (17.9 ± 6.4 ng/mg protein), while in the amnion the concentration fell to levels of the placental tissue (2.3 ± 1.9 and 1.4 ± 1.0 ng/mg protein, respectively). Pyromycin and cyclohexamide blocked Prl synthesis [50–52]. The difference was seen in culture and tissue content. Furthermore, it was demonstrated in such tissue cultures that incorporation of labeled amino acids occurred into Prl [50]. In a recent report [52], Prl release was found from the placenta and decidua. The release of Prl was three times higher than the tissue content of the hormone. Similar to a clinical study [349], bromoergocryptine did not modify Prl release into the culture medium [52]. The various data and the report by Golander et al. [351] indicate that the main source of Prl in amniotic fluid is the decidua. Immunocytochemical studies have confirmed this [427].

Recently, the capacity of human decidual tissue to synthesize Prl de novo was found to correlate with the levels of Prl in amniotic fluid [434]. Maximal concentrations of Prl in both amniotic fluid and samples of decidua were found prior to the 30th week of gestation and they declined simultaneously until term. A high correlation ($r = 0.90$, $P < 0.00005$) was found when the levels of Prl in amniotic fluid and the initial content of Prl in decidua from the same patient were compared. Also a very high correlation ($r = 0.96$, $P < 0.00005$) was seen between the ability of the decidua to produce Prl in vitro and the corresponding levels of Prl in amniotic fluid. Significant differences according to the sex of the fetus or the mode of delivery were absent. Rosenberg et al. [434] conclude that decidual tissue varies throughout late gestation in the initial content of Prl and its ability to synthesize Prl de novo, resulting in a high degree of correlation with Prl levels in amniotic

Table 114. Prolactin in normal human amniotic fluid

Weeks of gestation	Prl (ng/ml)	n	Ref.
20	2300	10	319
Term	350	5	
14–23	2577	7	325
29	500	1	349
36	468	1	
Term	437	5	277
32	775	18	352
12–20	365	179	347
21–30	481	70	
31–41	443	70	
Third trimester	745	58	348
12–22	1991	15	355
Third trimester	775	18	358
10	4.2	–	359
15–17	1314	–	
32–40	456	–	
16	1337	20	360
16–20	1803	32	361
36–39	931	33	362
40–43	885	35	
20	2215	10	363
Term	931	8	
9–16	37.6	9	129
38	150.5	7	
39	176.3	3	
40	177.1	8	
41	179.0	3	
42	128.0	6	

fluid and that the decidual tissue is the major source of amniotic fluid Prl. The role of such high levels of Prl in amniotic fluid seems to be osmoregulatory [352–354]. It was demonstrated [355] that addition of ovine Prl to the fetal side of human term amnion in vitro is associated with a decrease in membrane permeability to tritiated water. With increasing Prl concentration, the permeability was progressively impaired. The study results suggested that Prl acts predominantly on the differential flow rather than on bulk flow of water across the amnion [354].

Furthermore, Prl in amniotic fluid might be related to fetal lung maturity. A significant correlation between the L/S ratio and the Prl level in amniotic fluid was found [356] and is in agreement with studies on Prl levels in cord blood, indicating that fetal lung maturation and surfactant formation are functions of fetal Prl concentration [357]. Data on Prl in normal human amniotic fluid throughout gestation are summarized in Table 113. Besides the data listed in Table 114, Prl has also been measured throughout gestation by several other groups [364–366].

The course of Prl levels in human amniotic fluid throughout gestation differs from maternal and fetal blood. The Prl concentration in amniotic fluid is up to 100 times higher than in maternal or cord blood [319]. Prl in human amniotic fluid was detected after the 8th week of gestation [359, 365]. In one case at 8 weeks, no Prl was measurable [364]. A steep rise in concentration occurs with a maximum at 15–17 weeks of gestation [359]. Others

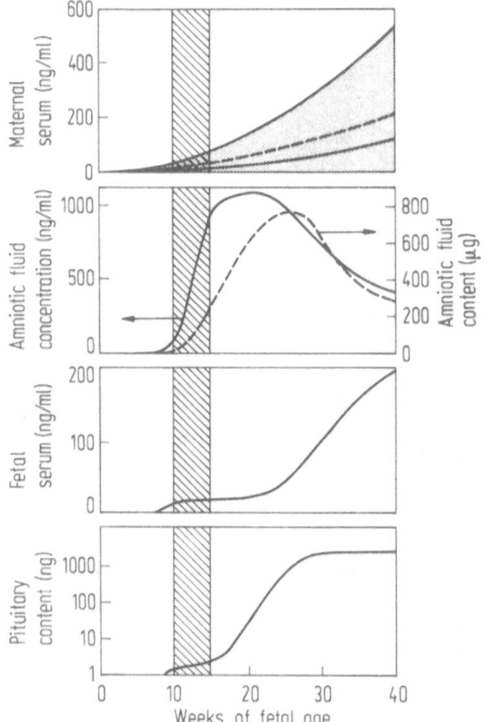

Fig. 16. Prolactin pattern throughout pregnancy in maternal serum, amniotic fluid, and fetal serum and pituitary. Prolactin content in amniotic fluid was derived from the observed concentrations multiplied by the estimated amniotic fluid volumes. The vertical *shaded area* represents the time of most rapid accumulation of prolactin in the amniotic fluid (10–15 weeks). (Clements et al. 1977 [359])

have found peak concentrations around 20 weeks of gestation [111, 347] or 22–26 weeks of gestation [365, 366]. A decrease toward term has been found in most of the studies [319, 359, 363–366] except for Biswas [347] who could not detect a significant difference between the values at 22–30 and 31–41 weeks of gestation. No major change was seen during the last weeks of gestation [129, 347, 359, 362, 364–366]. A wide range of values are present [364]. The changes of Prl in maternal and cord blood, fetal pituitary content, as well as in amniotic fluid concentration and content are presented in Fig. 16 [359]. The total amount of Prl in amniotic fluid continues to increase after the peak concentration in amniotic fluid has been reached because of the volume changes that occur after that time [350, 359].

A significant correlation ($P < 0.05$) has been found for amniotic fluid versus fetal pituitary content of Prl [359], but not for amniotic fluid versus pituitary concentration [359], amniotic fluid versus fetal blood [348, 349, 359], and amniotic fluid versus maternal blood [348, 349, 363]. Prl levels in amniotic fluid have been investigated in a number of pathologic conditions of pregnancy. In Rh incompatibility, a significantly higher Prl concentration ($P < 0.05$) in amniotic fluid has been reported [352]. In 25 cases with moderately severe or severe Rh incompatibility, a Prl level of 1,746 ng/ml was found while in normal cases the value was 775 ng/ml. In other studies, high or low [331] and normal levels were measured [129, 331, 347] even in cases of fetal death [331]. In pregnant women with diabetes mellitus (n = 19), the mean Prl level was also elevated when compared to controls [352]. Several studies have given data on Prl in patients with preeclampsia or essential hypertension [352, 358, 362]. The data are presented in Table 115.

In comparison, Prl levels in maternal blood were also found elevated in preeclampsia [352, 358] and significantly decreased ($P < 0.01$) in another report [362]. Definite conclusions cannot be drawn from these results.

In five cases with fetal intrauterine growth retardation, significantly higher values for Prl in amniotic fluid were measured than in normal cases [352].

Table 115. Prl in amniotic fluid in patients with preeclampsia or essential hypertension

Clinical diagnosis	Weeks of gestatior	n	Prl (ng/ml)	P[a]	Ref.
Normal	Third trimester	18	775		43, 358
Moderately to severe preeclampsia	Third trimester	14	2041	<0.05	
Normal	36–39	33	931	NS	362
Preeclampsia	36–39	14	1023		
Essential hypertension	36–39	10	583		
Normal	40–43	35	885		
Preeclampsia	40–43	9	736	NS	

[a] P, Significance between normal and abnormal conditions

A few cases have also been investigated in other pathologic conditions, such as anencephaly and spina bifida, hydramnios, intrauterine death, and cephalothoracopagus [179, 352, 362, 363]. Conclusive data were not obtained.

In the prenatal diagnosis of primary pituitary dysgenesis, low Prl concentration appears to be an indicator [360]. No major changes in the Prl level in amniotic fluid were seen under treatment with prostaglandin $F_{2\alpha}$ for induction of abortion up to 7 h [325, 355]. Chlorpromazine application was associated with a decrease of Prl in amniotic fluid and an increase in the maternal circulation [355], again pointing toward the independence of maternal Prl regulation and Prl in amniotic fluid. This is also reflected in the data obtained from a pregnancy treated with the prolactin inhibitor bromoergocryptine [349]. Maternal levels were suppressed and amniotic fluid levels unchanged. After intra-amniotic or intravenous injection of dehydroepiandrosterone sulfate, a rise in the maternal Prl level occurred, probably due to the increased levels of estrogens, but Prl concentrations in amniotic fluid did not reveal any consistent changes, leading to the conclusion that estrogens may not be implicated in the control of Prl in amniotic fluid [361].

VI. Adrenocorticotropic Hormone (ACTH)

Only a few data are available on ACTH in amniotic fluid [149, 367, 368]. The values throughout gestation are summarized in Table 116.

Table 116. ACTH in amniotic fluid throughout gestation [367]

Weeks of gestation	n	ACTH (pg/ml; mean ± SD)
10–18	15	208.7 ± 90.6
26–30	11	429.5 ± 180.4
31–32	12	201.3 ± 86.1
33–34	20	194.5 ± 129.4
35–36	17	163.6 ± 87.5
37–38	12	175.5 ± 54.4
39–40	16	170.9 ± 78.9
41–42	6	179.3 ± 46.7

At the time of delivery, Allen et al. [368] found a mean concentration of ACTH of 211 pg/ml (range 93–439 pg/ml). In another study, the concentrations before labor and at the end of the first stage of labor were compared, and an increase from 162.7 to 195.2 pg/ml was found [149]. Major differences of ACTH levels in amniotic fluid according to the sex of the fetus or due to various complications of pregnancy were not detected as seen in Table 117.

In a case of anencephaly, a low level (20 pg/ml) was measured [368], and in a case with Nelson syndrome, serial measurements were done in maternal and fetal blood as well as in amniotic fluid as listed in Table 118.

The origin of ACTH in amniotic fluid is most likely the fetal urine since the concentration in amniotic fluid more closely resembles fetal than maternal

Table 117. Effect of sex of the fetus, uterine activity, and various complications of pregnancy on the ACTH concentration in human amniotic fluid [367]

Clinical diagnosis		n	ACTH (pg/ml; mean ± SD)
Fetal sex	Male	52	176.7 ± 89.8
	Female	27	166.9 ± 112.2
Normal pregnancy		16	143.3 ± 49.7
Uterine activity		18	196.8 ± 125.0
Rh disease		10	158.7 ± 78.6
Hypertension		17	153.1 ± 56.2
Diabetes		11	208.6 ± 154.1
Hydramnios		4	156.0 ± 45.1
Jaundice of pregnancy		5	145.4 ± 38.5

Table 118. ACTH during pregnancy in a patient with Nelson syndrome [368]

	ACTH (pg/ml)		
	Maternal plasma	Amniotic fluid	Fetal plasma
Before pregnancy	5240	–	–
3 Months	2600	20	–
6 Months	7230	110	–
Term	21200	221	–
Delivery	23400	–	714

ACTH concentration [368]. For instance, similar trends of ACTH concentration in fetal cord blood and amniotic fluid have been reported [367, 369]. Furthermore, there is quite a high ACTH level in the first urine of the newborn, which closely approximates that in the amniotic fluid [367]. Transport of ACTH across the placenta does not occur [368–370]. So far, ACTH determinations in amniotic fluid have not been used for clinical evaluations.

VII. Human Growth Hormone (HGH)

HGH was first described in 1969 [371]. In the meantime, only few reports have followed [316, 319, 365, 372]. The results of HGH determinations in normal amniotic fluid are listed in Table 119.

Single data and mean values of HGH are also demonstrated in Fig. 17. Similarities between somatomedin and Prl in amniotic fluid are shown. Correlations between HGH, somatomedin, and Prl in amniotic fluid are highly significant: $P < 0.001$ [365].

In comparison to maternal levels, the concentration in amniotic fluid in early pregnancy is similar. However, at term the the HGH values in amniotic fluid are 10% of the maternal values [316]. Compared to the fetal blood levels in the first half of pregnancy, the values of HGH in amniotic fluid are 6% of the fetal concentration and at term only 1% [316]. These data indicate that HGH increases in amniotic fluid in early pregnancy until the second trimester [316, 365]. Thereafter, a continuous decrease was found [316, 365]. Only Tyson et al. [319] found higher values at term than at 20 weeks of gestation (Table 116). In a pregnancy with bromoergocryptine therapy, HGH did not change markedly from 29 to 36 weeks of gestation (16.2 and 13.7 ng/ml,

Table 119. HGH in normal human amniotic fluid

Weeks of gestation	n	HGH (ng/ml; mean)	Ref.
30–40	5	6.4	372
20	10	10.0	319
Term	7	30.0	
11	1	0.2	316
20–28	7	2.7	
32–41	13	1.0	
42–43	7	0.2	

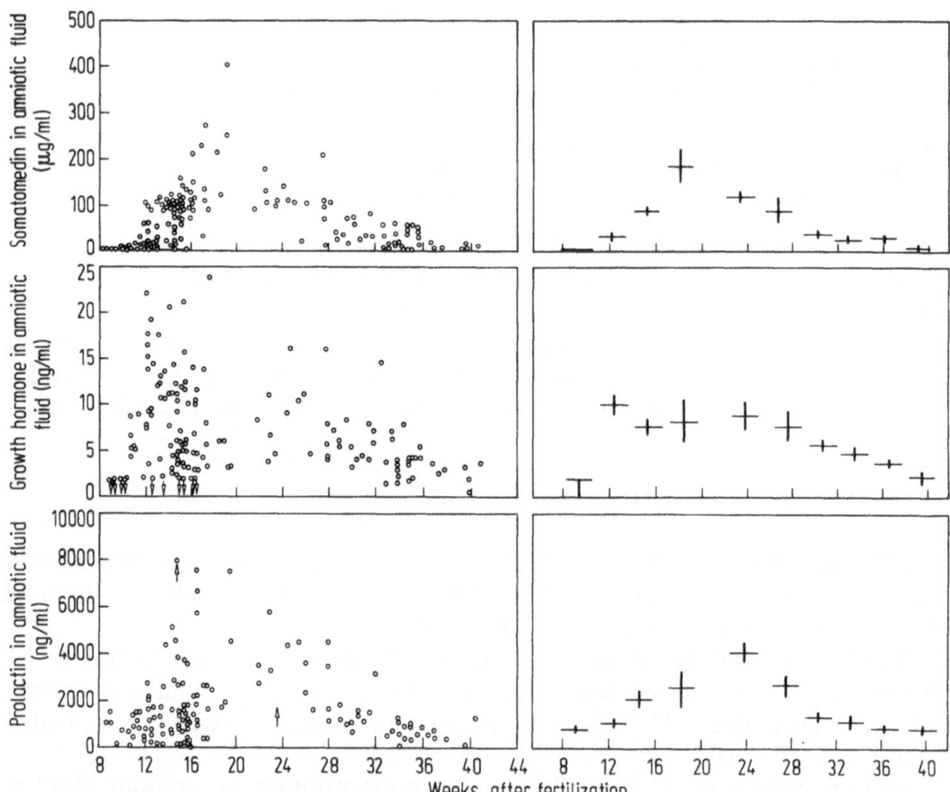

Fig. 17. Amniotic fluid somatomedin reactivity, growth hormone, and prolactin levels at different gestational ages. Individual data are shown on the *left* and the means ± SEM, grouped in 3-week periods, are shown on the *right*. ↑ greater than; ↓ less than. (Chochinov et al. 1976 [365])

respectively) [349]. HGH does not cross the placenta, but clearance from amniotic fluid is similar to other proteins [35]. Most of this clearance is due to fetal swallowing [35].

In abnormal pregnancies, such as postmaturity, hydramnios, Rh isoimmunization, ABO incompatibility, and cephalothoracopagus, similar concentrations were measured [179, 316, 372]. In three cases of fetal death in utero, a high HGH activity (20.7–41.0 ng/ml) was found [372]. It is most likely that HGH in amniotic fluid is of fetal origin since there is an increase of HGH in the fetal circulation first and a decrease toward term [316, 373]. Further clinical data are lacking.

VIII. Somatomedin and Somatomedin C

Available data indicate that somatomedin plays an important role in fetal growth [374]. In term human amniotic fluid, somatomedin activity (SMA) was measured by a rat cartilage bioassay, and a mean activity of 0.07 U/ml was found [375]. It is present in several stable molecule sizes [375]. Studies throughout pregnancy by these assay procedures showed an increase of the activity toward term as listed in Table 120 [376]. In normal term pregnancies, SMA in amniotic fluid was lower than in the maternal blood and fetal blood [376].

Table 120. Somatomedin activity (SMA) in human amniotic fluid [376]

Weeks of gestation	n	SMA (U/ml; mean ± SEM)	P[a]
12–16	12	0.04 ± 0.01	
33–36	6	0.09 ± 0.01	<0.05
Term	41	0.07 ± 0.01	<0.01

[a] P, Significance of sex differences

For somatomedin C, a radioreceptor assay was utilized [365]. In amniotic fluid, the rise in growth hormone precedes the increase of somatomedin C activity [365]. The comparison is shown in Fig. 18. The fall in amniotic fluid concentration of this protein is thought to be due to the fetal renal maturation as evidenced by a rise in the creatinine concentration and a decrease in protein concentration in amniotic fluid [365]. The negative correlation between creatinine and somatomedin C, growth hormone, and Prl in amniotic fluid is highly significant: $P < 0.001$ [365].

IX. Thyroid-Stimulating Hormone (TSH)

In contrast to the increasing levels of TSH in maternal and cord blood during pregnancy, undetectable or low levels have been reported in amniotic fluid [316, 377–380]. The data are listed in Table 121. In a pregnancy with a cephalothoracopagus, the TSH concentration was found to be 4.0 μU/ml at 28 weeks of gestation [179].

Differences have been noted using bioassay and radioimmunoassay [377]. While with the bioassay higher levels of TSH in human amniotic fluid were found when compared to the adult serum (0.8 versus 0.36 mU/ml), the reverse was found with a radioimmunoassay [377]. The possibility of using TSH measurement in amniotic fluid for intrauterine detection of fetal hypothyroidism has not yet been exploited [379].

Table 121. TSH in human amniotic fluid

Weeks of gestation	n	TSH (μU/ml)	Ref.
11	1	1.2	316
20–28	7	1.4	
32–41	13	1.2	
42–43	7	1.3	
16–42	20	–[a]	378
–	–	–[b]	381

[a] Below the sensitivity level of the method (3.7 μU/ml)
[b] Undetectable up to 2.8 μU/ml

X. Thyroid Hormones

1. Thyroxine (T_4)

Thyroxine in human amniotic fluid was detected as early as 10–12 weeks of gestation [382, 383]. Throughout gestation an increase in concentration is measurable [378, 380, 384, 385]. A correlation coefficient of r = 0.533 between T_4 in amniotic fluid and gestational age was found: $P < 0.005$ [384]. Others noted relatively constant PBJ or T_4 concentrations in amniotic fluid during gestation [385, 386] or even a decrease in T_4 concentration [382]. Recently, it was calculated that from 10–30 weeks of gestation, T_4 increases in human amniotic fluid significantly ($P < 0.01$), reaching a peak concentration at 25–30 weeks of gestation, followed by a significant decrease ($P < 0.01$) toward term as demonstrated in Fig. 18 [383]. Data on T_4 are summarized in Table 122.

The relationship of total and free T_4 in amniotic fluid, maternal blood, and cord blood is shown in Table 123. Correlations between total and free T_4 in amniotic fluid, maternal blood, or cord blood are not present [384].

Most of the T_4 in amniotic fluid appears to be bound to protein since up to 99.7% is nondialyzable [384, 389], but the dialyzable fraction is increased when compared to serum levels in euthyroid adults [389].

In gestational diabetes at 36–40 weeks, a T_4 concentration of 0.59 μg/100 ml was found, and in intrauterine malnutrition at 31–35 weeks, the T_4 level in amniotic fluid was 0.6 μg/100 ml [388]. Suggestion has been made to use T_4 by in utero administration to treat the hypothyroid fetus to minimize irreversable mental retardation [387, 390], to reduce the size of fetal goiter [182], and to enhance fetal lung maturity [391, 392].

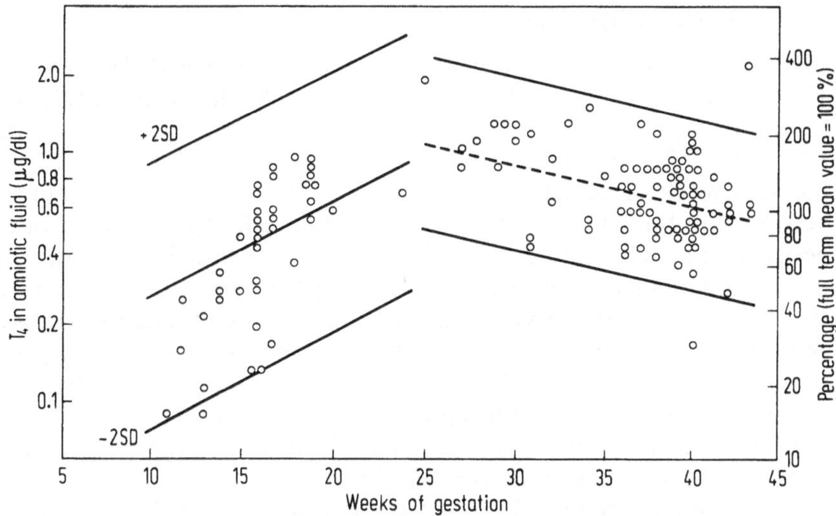

Fig. 18. T_4 concentrations in amniotic fluid versus gestational age. The *vertical axis* on the *left* is on a logarithmic scale; on the *right*, T_4 values are indicated on a logarithmic scale; ±2SD from the regression line are also indicated. (Klein et al. 1980 [383])

Table 122. T_4 in human amniotic fluid

Weeks of gestation	n	T_4 (µg/100 ml)	Ref.
16–20	38	0.46	382
30–42	71	0.38	
15–29	19	0.39	378
20–30	2	0.51	
31–35	7	0.31	
36–42	26	0.44	
<20	11	0.24	384
38–40	18	0.62	
Term	5	0.25	387
15–19	17	0.26	380
20–30	3	0.27	
36–42	29	0.31	
12–19	18	0.22	388
31–35	49	0.55	
36–40	52	0.51	

Table 123. Total and free T_4 concentration (µg/100 ml) in human amniotic fluid, cord blood, and maternal blood

	Amniotic fluid	Cord blood	Maternal blood	Ref.
Total T_4	0.64	11.25	9.31	384
Total T_4	0.54	9.4	10.8	389
Free T_4	4.13	2.56	2.67	384

2. 3,3′,5-Triiodothyronine (T_3)

In four studies, T_3 was described as undetectable with less than 25, 15, or 12.5 ng/100 ml, respectively [378, 384, 380, 388]. More recently, the concentration of T_3 in amniotic fluid in five pregnancies at term was found to be 8.6 ng/ml [387]; in concentrated amniotic fluid, T_3 was detected as early as the 12th week of gestation [387]. Thereafter, T_3 was measured in 15 samples between the 16th and 20th weeks of gestation at 9.4 ng/100 ml and in 45 samples between the 30th and 42nd weeks of gestation at 5.8 ng/100 ml. There were huge standard errors, and therefore the apparent decrease was not statistically significant [382]. Higher values (30 ng/ml) have been found by others after concentration procedures [389]. Recently, the study by Klein et al. [383] showed low levels at 10–15 weeks of gestation (3.6 ng/100 ml), followed by a progressive and significant increase throughout gestation (10.8 ng/100 ml) as shown in Fig. 19. A comparison of T_3 in amniotic fluid to maternal blood and umbilical cord blood levels is summarized in Table 124.

Only a small amount (1.7%) of the hormone is dialyzable [389], but this is increased when compared to the serum of euthyroid adults: therefore, the percent of dialyzable T_3 and also T_4 was suggested to be potentially useful for establishing the diagnosis of congenital hypothyroidism before birth [389].

Table 124. Triiodothyronine (T_3) concentration (ng/100 ml) in human amniotic fluid, cord blood, and maternal blood

Amniotic fluid	Cord blood	Maternal blood	Ref.
<15	55	201	384
30	30	150	389

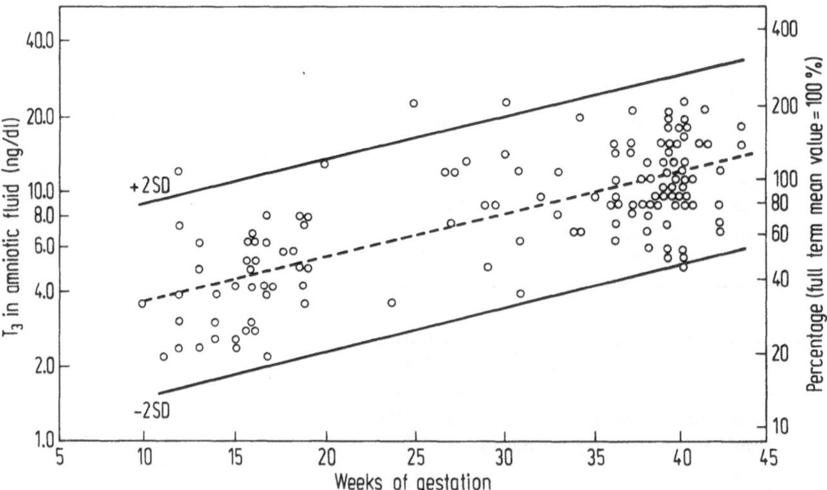

Fig. 19. T_3 concentrations in amniotic fluid versus gestational age. The *vertical axis* on the *left* is on a logarithmic scale; on the *right*, T_3 values are indicated on a logarithmic scale; ± 2 SD from the regression line are also indicated. (Klein et al. 1980 [383])

3. Reverse 3,3′,5′-Triiodothyronine (rT_3)

Several studies reported on rT_3 in amniotic fluid. Most of the investigators described a decrease of rT_3 in amniotic fluid throughout gestation [378, 381, 386, 388, 389]. In some studies, an increase of rT_3 was found [380]. Possible influences of the assay techniques are considered [380]. In a recent study [383], it was demonstrated that rT_3 increases significantly from 10 to 20 weeks

Table 125. rT_3 concentration in human amniotic fluid

Weeks of gestation	n	rT_3 (ng/ml)	Ref.	Weeks of gestation	n	rT_3 (ng/ml)	Ref.
20	21	330	378	12–19	18	159	388
20–30	4	323		31–35	49	66	
31–35	7	95		36–40	52	59	
36–42	23	93		Term	5	43	387
Term	9	82	389	Term	4	22–82	
21–25	6	353	381	10	2	76	380
26–30	7	131		15–19	17	80	
31–35	14	94		20–30	5	52	
36–40	20	93		36–42	30	143	

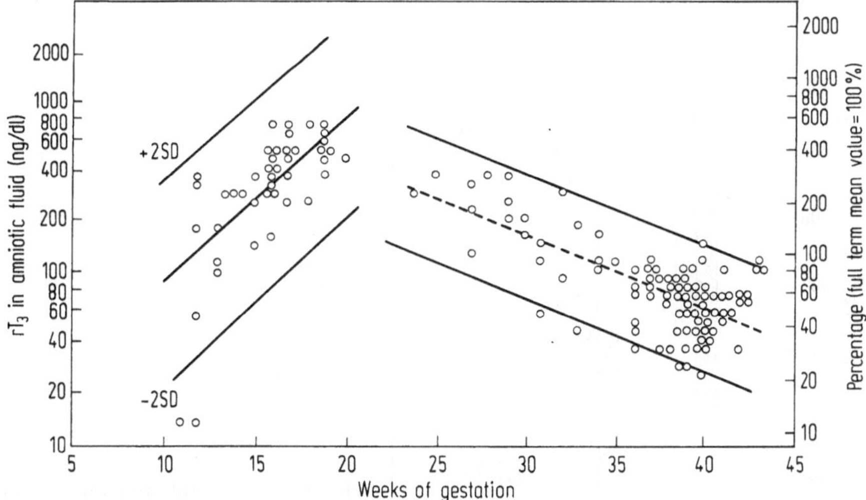

Fig. 20. rT_3 concentrations in amniotic fluid versus gestational age. The *vertical axis* on the *left* is on a logarithmic scale; on the *right*, rT_3 values are indicated on a logarithmic scale; ±2 SD from the regression line are also indicated. (Klein et al. 1980 [383])

of gestation ($P < 0.01$). A peak concentration is reached at 17–20 weeks of gestation, and a significant decrease ($P < 0.01$) follows toward term as illustrated in Fig. 20. The other available data are listed in Table 125.

The proposal to identify pregnancies of less than 30 weeks of gestation by rT_3 measurements [378] is not supported by later studies [381, 388]. In complicated pregnancies, rT_3 concentrations in amniotic fluid were not significantly different from those observed in normal pregnancies of the same gestational age [381]. However, in pregnant patients with severe Rh isoimmunization, the values for rT_3 were significantly higher ($P < 0.05$) as demonstrated in Fig. 21. Good correlation of rT_3 in amniotic fluid and optical density (ΔOD 450) was found [381]. Others [386] could not detect differences for rT_3 in pregnancies without severely affected fetuses.

No correlation was seen with the lecithin/sphingomyelin ratio [381], while in one study a significant ($P < 0.01$) negative correlation was noted [386]. It appears that rT_3 might be useful in the detection of fetal hypothyroidism in utero [378, 388, 393]. Differences of opinion have been raised [380]. The intrauterine detection of fetal hypothyroidism is of interest since an effective therapy appears possible by intra-amniotic injection of T_4 [182, 387, 390, 394]. The data of such a study [387] are given in Table 126.

This leads not only to an increase of T_4 in the amniotic fluid but also in the fetal circulation, indicating effective absorption of T_4 from amniotic fluid [387, 394]. The high levels of T_3 and rT_3 concentration in amniotic fluid after the injection of T_4 might be due to amniotic membrane metabolism of T_4 and may explain the high T_3 concentration found in amniotic fluid in early gestation when levels of T_4 and most likely rT_3 in fetal serum are low [387]. The effectiveness of such prenatal intrauterine therapeutic approaches has also been demonstrated by others, showing the suitability of rT_3 measure-

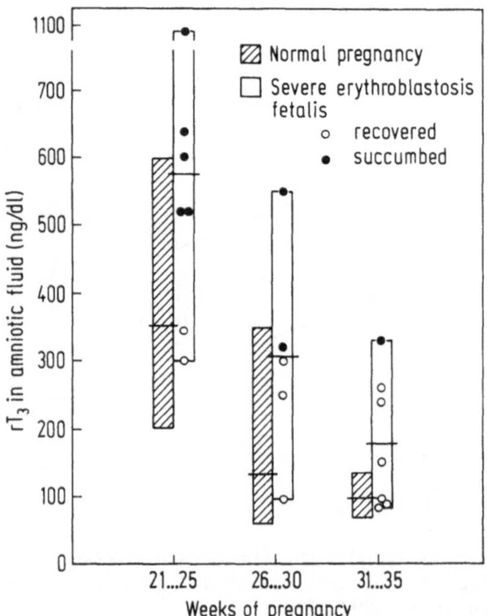

Fig. 21. rT_3 concentrations in amniotic fluid from 19 patients with severe erythroblastosis fetalis compared to normal pregnancy (mean and range) at 21–25 and 31–35 weeks of gestation. (Osathanondh et al. 1978 [381])

ments in amniotic fluid [395]. However, doubts were recently raised regarding the use of rT_3 measurements in amniotic fluid as a reliable tool for diagnosing intrauterine fetal hypothyriodism [396].

Table 126. Iodothyronine concentration in human amniotic fluid and cord blood after intra-amniotic injection of T_4 [387]

	T_4 (μg/100 ml)	T_3 (ng/100 ml)	rT_3 (ng/100 ml)
Amniotic fluid			
Pre T_4 injection	0.25	8.6	43.4
Post T_4 injection	12.6	113.0	1238
Cord blood			
Pre T_4 injection	10.3	48.3	254.0
Post T_4 injection	27.2	61.3	657.0

4. 3,3′-Diiodothyronine (T_2)

This iodothyronine has been measured in amniotic fluid throughout normal gestation. There was a rise of T_2 from 4.1 ng/100 ml at 15–16 weeks of gestation to 10.9 ng/100 ml at term [397]. In another study, the level of T_2 at term was found to be 20 compared to 27 ng/100 ml in the corresponding blood samples from the mother and 20 ng/100 ml in the cord blood [389]. It appears that T_2 is derived from deiodination of T_3 and rT_3 [397]. The clinical usefulness of T_2 measurements in amniotic fluid for the evaluation of fetal hypothyroidism needs to be studied.

5. 3′,5′-Diiodothyronine and 3,5-Diiodothyronine

Both diiodothyronines have been measured by RIA in amniotic fluid [428–430]. The available data are summarized in Table 127.

The values during the last trimester for 3′,5′-diiodothyronine are similar in both studies [428, 424]. However, in one investigation [428], in 9 of 19 samples the hormone was undetectable (< 2 ng/100 ml). Results in cases with abnormal fetal thyroid function have not yet been reported so far.

Table 127. 3′,5′-Diiodothyronine and 3,5-diiodothyronine concentration in human amniotic fluid

Weeks of gestation	n	Thyroid hormone	Concentration (ng/100 ml; mean ± SEM)	Ref.
Term	10	3′,5′-diiodothyronine	5.4 ± 1.0	428
15–20	9	3′,5′-diiodothyronine	15.2 ± 1.6	429
33–40	8		5.8 ± 0.6	
33–44	14	3,5-diiodothyronine	0.9 ± 0.7	430

6. 3′-Monoiodothyronine (3′-T_1)

Recently, a radioimmunoassay for 3′-T_1 was developed [431]. The mean concentration (± SD) in amniotic fluid (n = 20) was 17.6 ± 6.7 ng/100 ml at 15–20 weeks of gestation and 12.3 ± 3.6 ng/100 ml (n = 12) at 33–40 weeks of gestation. These values were significantly different ($P < 0.001$) and higher than in the adult serum ($P < 0.001$). It is concluded that these high values are not due to cross reactivity of 3,3′-T_2, 3′,5′-T_2, 3,5-T_2, or rT_3 in the 3′-T_1 RIA since the concentrations of these hormones are too low in amniotic fluid [378, 387, 389, 397, 428, 429, 430] to influence 3′-T_1 measurements [431].

XI. Parathyroid Hormone (PTH)

Only few data have been published so far [432]. In amniotic fluid obtained at term at the time of cesarian section a range of values between 347 and 861 ng/ml and a level of 4.3 to 6.6 mg/100 ml calcium was found. In one case with maternal hyperparathyroidism the amniotic fluid PTH-level at 34 weeks gestation was 253 pg/ml and the calcium concentration was 17.1 mg/100 ml. This indicates that parathyroid function of the mother changes the PTH and calcium levels in the fetus as reflected by the amniotic fluid values.

XII. Oxytocin

With the availability of a radioimmunoassay for oxytocin, this protein hormone was quantitated in amniotic fluid. Oxytocin was not detectable in all amniotic fluid samples investigated. Measurable levels were found in 89.7% [398]. There is a rise of oxytocin concentration in amniotic fluid from 7.8 ± 3.6 (SEM) pg/ml at 14–15 weeks of gestation to 43.9 ± 14.7 pg/ml at 40 weeks and 30.8 ± 10.5 pg/ml at 41–42 weeks [398]. In 8 of 11 patients who had cesarean section after the onset of labor, the oxytocin concentration ranged 1.0–90.6 pg/ml. In three of ten patients who had cesarean section without labor, the level was 4.6, 51.9, and 60.0 pg/ml, respectively [399]. Seppälä et al. [400] reported higher levels. In 12 women during late pregnancy without uterine contraction, the values varied between 150 and 800 pg/ml (medium 275 pg/ml), and in 18 women in labor the concentration ranged 110–1,600 pg/ml (medium 695 pg/ml). This difference is statistically significant ($P < 0.01$).

Amniotic fluid samples contaminated with meconium contained 1,000 to 1,400 pg/ml of oxytocin. The highest values were found in the samples most heavily contaminated with meconium. In meconium, oxytocin was quantitated as high as 175,000 pg/g wet weight and in first voided urine from newborns the values ranged 1,800–2,800 pg/ml.

The source of oxytocin in amniotic fluid is normally fetal urine. Since the ratio of amniotic fluid and fetal urine for oxytocin is 2:1, other sources must exist. Umbilical arterial oxytocin concentration is higher than in amniotic fluid, particularly in labor. Therefore, there could also be diffusion or transfer from the umbilical cord or the placenta into the amniotic fluid [398, 399].

Oxytocin in amniotic fluid appears to be biologically inactive in more than 90% of cases [400].

XIII. Glucagon

Glucagon was first measured in amniotic fluid by Gerlini et al. [401] using RIA. The study was done in 15 normal pregnant women having amniocentesis between the 37th and 40th weeks of gestation and in 28 pregnant women with Rh isoimmunization with 51 amniocenteses between the 25th and 39th weeks of gestation. The values of glucagon were similar to those in cord arterial plasma and maternal plasma [401]. The data at term are shown in Table 128 in comparison to the glucose and immunoreactive insulin levels. Changes during pregnancy could also be determined in Rh isoimmunization. The data are illustrated in Fig. 22.

Table 128. Immunoreactive glucagon (IRG), immunoreactive insulin (IRI), and glucose in amniotic fluid in normal pregnant women and patients with Rh isoimmunization at term [401]

		Normal	n	Rh iso-immunization	n
IRG	(pg/ml)[a]	59.0 ± 12.7	15	63.0 ± 12.0	13
IRI	(μU/ml)[a]	7.6 ± 1.2	14	8.8 ± 1.6	14
Glucose	(mg/100 ml)[a]	8.4 ± 2.1	15	9.7 ± 2.1	13

[a] Mean ± SEM

At 25–28 weeks of gestation, IRG was detected in all cases with a subsequent increase that was significant after 32 weeks and a decrease after 37 weeks of gestation. Correlation with the optical density change at 450 nm of the amniotic fluid was not found. The levels of IRG in amniotic fluid and maternal plasma were similar in both the control group and the patients with Rh isoimmunization. The content of IRG in amniotic fluid is most likely fetal in origin since IRG was present in the first voided neonatal urine and does not pass across the placenta from the mother to the fetus [401]. At least for moderate Rh isoimmunzation, no differences from normal are measurable. In early pregnancy (16–18 weeks), values for glucagon in amniotic fluid were also reported by Pearlman and Gordin [402] to be 47 ± 18 pg/ml (mean ± SD), which are similar to those reported by Gerlini et al. [401] at 25–32 weeks of gestation in Rh-isoimmunized pregnancies. A significant ($P < 0.05$) increase of glucagon in amniotic fluid throughout gestation was shown by Sperling et al. who measured a concentration at 10–20 weeks of gestation of 43 pg/ml and at 30–40 weeks of gestation of 117 pg/ml. In this study, glucagon in amniotic fluid failed to predict neonatal glucose homeostasis. Investigations of the nature of glucagon in amniotic fluid revealed that most of the glucagon was not the biologically active compound with a molecular weight of 3,500 [403]. A correlation of glucose, insulin, and glucagon in amniotic fluid was not detectable [402].

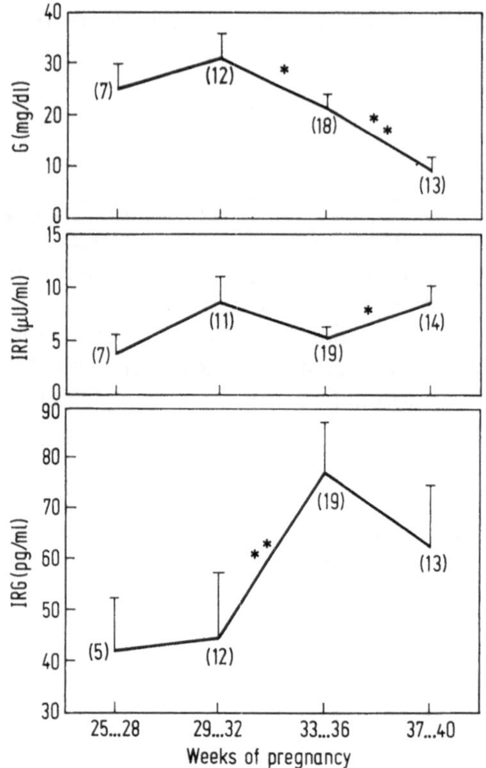

Fig. 22. Changes of glucose *(G)*, immunoreactive insulin *(IRI)*, and immunoreactive glucagon (IRG) in the amniotic fluid of rhesus isoimmunized pregnancies at various states of gestation. The number of patients are in ***parentheses***. ***Asterisks*** indicate statistically significant differences. (Gerlini et al. 1977 [401])

The usefulness of glucagon measurements for prenatal diagnosis of inborn errors of carbohydrate metabolism, such as glucagon storage disease type I and pancreatic endocrinopathies such as familial hyperinsulinemia, has not yet been elucidated.

XIV. Insulin

Insulin in amniotic fluid was first reported in 1969 [331, 371]. Subsequently, several publications have evaluated insulin levels in amniotic fluid in normal and complicated pregnancies.

Between 13 and 16 weeks of gestation, the values are less than 5 μU/ml and are therefore below the sensitivity of the method for exact calculation [404]. During this time, the insulin content of amniotic fluid changes from about 1 to 2 μU/ml. At 17 weeks of gestation, the mean concentration increases to 4.8 μU/ml [404]. The data are listed in Table 129 and Fig. 23.

There is an increase of insulin in amniotic fluid throughout gestation [401, 404], which is slight but significant, ($P < 0.02$) [405]. Others have found an increase up to 34 weeks and thereafter a marked decrease [406].

Differences according to the sex of the fetus were not found [407]. There is a significant relationship between insulin content in amniotic fluid measured 1 day before delivery and infant birth weight ($P < 0.02$) [405]. Furthermore,

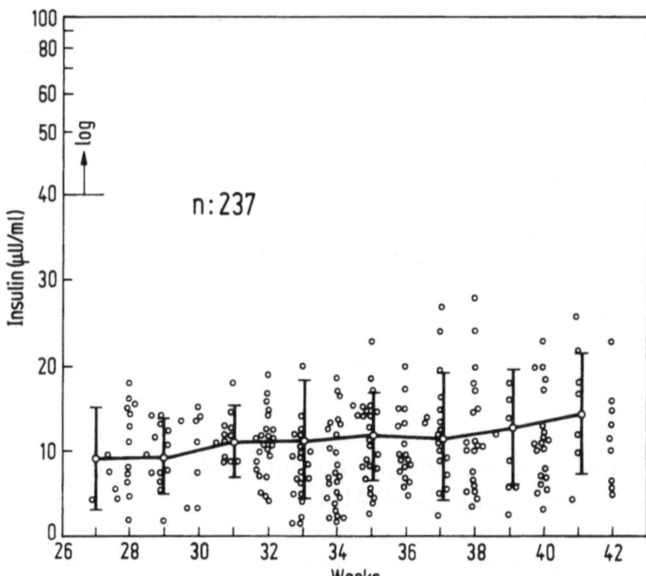

Fig. 23. Insulin concentrations in amniotic fluid in normal pregnancies; individual values, means, and SD. (Weiss 1979 [404])

Table 129. Insulin in human amniotic fluid

Weeks of gestation	n	Insulin (μU/ml)	Ref.
17	13	4.8	404
18–20	3	6.7	
21–22	2	7.8	
23–24	2	4.9	
25–26	2	7.9	
27–28	–	8.3	
41–42	–	13.3	
37–40	15	7.6	401
38–40	6	11.3	411

a significant correlation ($P<0.001$) was obtained between insulin levels in amniotic fluid and neonatal glucose disappearance. Newborn low blood glucose (less than 20 ng/100 ml) developed significantly ($P<0.001$) more often when insulin concentration in amniotic fluid was above 100 μU/ml [408]. Therefore, insulin measurements in amniotic fluid might be used for prediction of neonatal hypoglycemia [408].

Maternal weight gain above 12 kg leads to significantly elevated maternal insulin levels but also to a significant elevation of insulin in cord blood and amniotic fluid [407]. This is confirmed by a further study [409] as indicated in Table 130.

Similar effects on insulin in all three compartments were also induced by maternal glucose infusion [407]. The relation of insulin levels in fetal blood and amniotic fluid to maternal carbohydrate metabolism is also reflected in

Table 130. Effect of maternal weight gain on insulin concentration

	Insulin (μU/ml; mean ± SEM)				P[a]	Ref.
	Weight gain < 12 kg	n	Weight gain > 12 kg	n		
Amniotic fluid	5.0 ± 0.4	19	11.2 ± 1.1	5	>0.001	407
Fetal blood	9.8 ± 0.4	19	19.9 ± 4.3	5	>0.001	
Maternal blood	23.9 ± 0.5	19	38.4 ± 1.8	5	>0.001	
Amniotic fluid	6.0 ± 0.4	20	12.2 ± 1.1	15	>0.001	409
Fetal blood	10.8 ± 0.4	20	20.9 ± 3.3	15	>0.001	
Maternal blood	24.9 ± 0.5	20	39.4 ± 1.8	15	>0.001	

[a] P, Significance

changes of intrauterine insulin levels when pregnant women are treated with β-mimetic drugs [404, 410].

In one study an inverse relationship between amniotic fluid insulin levels and fetal lung maturity expressed by the L/S-ratio or lecithin/palmitic acid concentration was noted [406]. Insulin levels below 8 μU/ml were nearly always associated with mature levels of lecithin [406].

Sixty-six insulin determinations in amniotic fluid under tocolytic therapy between the 27th and 37th weeks of gestation showed a rise of insulin in amniotic fluid of 30% above the normal mean [404].

In pregnant diabetic women, insulin levels in amniotic fluid were found to be elevated [404, 410, 412]. In such conditions, it appears that the insulin levels in amniotic fluid reflect the level in the fetus [412] since insulin in amniotic fluid is mainly dependent on fetal urinary excretion [404]. In 38 cases of diabetic women with a classification of B–D [404], all insulin values were above normal. The mean concentration at 28 weeks of gestation was 38 μU/ml (4.2 times above normal) and at 38 weeks of gestation 215 μU/ml (1 time. above normal).

It was demonstrated that monitoring insulin values in amniotic fluid could considerably improve the outcome of pregnancies complicated by maternal diabetes [404, 410, 413]; insulin levels in amniotic fluid above 20 μU/ml indicate individuals who are more than White class A diabetic patients [414].

Differences in results are reported in pregnancies complicated by severe Rh isoimmunization. Weiss [404] demonstrated that in severe cases low normal insulin values are present, while Vidnes and Finne [415] found significantly ($P < 0.01$) higher levels in severely immunized women (Liley zone II and III). In moderately affected pregnancies, no difference was noted when compared to normal pregnancies [401].

In pregnancies complicated by preeclampsia, particularly when fetal growth retardation is present, the insulin levels in amniotic fluid were below the mean normal values [404].

In cases with fetal death in utero, essentially no insulin could be detected in amniotic fluid, pointing toward the fetus as the main source for this hormone in amniotic fluid [404, 411, 416]. In four cases with anencephalic fetuses, the insulin level in amniotic fluid was 10.0 ± 1.4 μg/ml, which is comparable to values found in normal pregnancies [416].

Regarding fetal lung maturation, an increased relationship between lecithin and insulin in amniotic fluid after 34–35 weeks of gestation was found; it was speculated that insulin might inhibit lecithin synthesis [406], while in another study no correlation between amniotic fluid values and the lecithin-sphingomyelin ratio was apparent [414]. Intravenous glucose administration to the mother did not change the insulin levels in amniotic fluid, while glucose concentration in amniotic fluid increased. Therefore, it was concluded that the insulin in human amniotic fluid is of fetal origin [416].

XV. Hypothalamic-Releasing Hormones

1. Thyrotropin-Releasing Hormone (TRH)

Isolation of TRH in human amniotic fluid was reported in 1974 [417]. The quantitation of TRH in human amniotic fluid by radioimmunoassay developed by Bassini and Utinger [418] was done recently by Morley et al. [386]. Before 32 weeks of gestation, a concentration of 169 pg/ml was found, which increased to 308 pg/ml for amniotic fluid specimens after 32 weeks of gestation, a significant increase ($P < 0.025$) [386]. In amniotic fluid from 23 pregnancies past 32 weeks, low TRH levels were more common in pregnancies with delivery of depressed newborns [386]. The data are listed in Table 131. A correlation of TRH in amniotic fluid with the L/S ratio, T_4, or rT_3 was not found [386].

Table 131. TRH levels in human amniotic fluid and Apgar score of the newborns [386]

		TRH (pg/ml)	P[a]
1-min Apgar score	<7	96	>0.01
	>7	315	
5-min Apgar score	<7	106	<0.05
	>7	290	

[a] P, Significance

2. Luteinizing Hormone-Releasing Hormone (LH-RH)

LH-RH was isolated and described to be present in considerable amounts in human amniotic fluid [417]. Further studies are lacking.

XVI. Neurophysin

In human amniotic fluid, neurophysin was measured by a heterologous RIA with antiserum to bovine neurophysin I. [419] In patients undergoing therapeutic abortions between the 3rd and 5th months of pregnancy, the neurophysin content of amniotic fluid was 14.4 ± 7.2 (SD) ng/ml. There was no significant difference between the 3rd, 4th, or 5th months (15.0, 13.9, and 15.7 ng/ml, respectively). These values are higher than the concentration found in plasma at the same stage of gestation [419].

XVII. β-Endorphin and "Humoral Endorphin"

This peptide was quantitated in human amniotic fluid by a double antibody RIA in 18 women after 36 weeks of gestation [420]. In 14 cases with clear amniotic fluid and a normal term delivery, the concentration of β-endorphin in amniotic fluid was 295 ± 72 pg/ml (mean ± SD). The other four cases with fetal distress had β-endorphin concentrations in amniotic fluid between 610 and 5,750 pg/ml [420].

In another study, β-endorphin was measured with a highly sensitive and specific homologous RIA at a lower concentration [421]. In six pregnancies at term, the level of β-endorphin in amniotic fluid was 104 ± 6 (SEM) pg/ml, and the simultaneously measured concentrations in cord blood and maternal blood were 250 ± 54 and 248 ± 28 pg/ml, respectively [421]. The significance of these findings remains to be determined.

Similarly, an enkephaline–like substance "humoral endorphin" was quantitated by RIA and compared with the levels in maternal and cord blood. The data are listed in Table 132 [435].

Table 132. Humoral endorphin in human amniotic fluid, umbilical cord blood, and maternal blood [435]

Weeks of gestation	Endorphin (leu-encephalin equivalents; mean ± SEM)					
	Amniotic fluid	n	Cord blood	n	Maternal blood	n
16–28	7.72 ± 0.42	12	15.39 ± 1.04	24	15.20 ± 1.61	4
38–42	5.90 ± 0.23	20	14.16 ± 0.65	22	14.99 ± 0.99	15

The levels in amniotic fluid are significantly lower than in maternal and cord blood. The molecular size of this compound renders it unlikely to pass the placenta. Therefore, the material in amniotic fluid is most likely fetal or placental in origin. The decrease in concentration as pregnancy advances could indicate increased disposition or metabolism and probably reflect fetal maturation [435].

XVIII. β-Melanocyte-Stimulating Hormone (β-MSH)

β-MSH has been quantitated by RIA in human amniotic fluid [422]. The levels in amniotic fluid are higher than in the maternal circulation and on the average above the concentration in cord blood (amniotic fluid = 612 pg/ml, fetal cord blood = 449 pg/ml, maternal serum = 246 pg/ml). Before 31 weeks of gestation, this hormone could not be detected in amniotic fluid. The available data are listed in Table 133.

Table 133. Concentration of β-MSH in human amniotic fluid [422]

Weeks of gestation	n	β-MSH (pg/ml)
23	1	0
26	1	0
32	2	350
36	4	543
37	2	519
38	2	1200
39	1	2025
43	1	300
44	2	1181

XIX. Conclusions

The previous chapters represent an up-to-date account of hormones in human amniotic fluid in normal and abnormal conditions. The methods of identification and quantitation are particularly detailed for steroids. It becomes obvious that many of the measured hormones have been determined in only a few instances. Data on the normal range at different stages of gestation throughout pregnancy under normal and pathological circumstances are often rare or absent and therefore the clinical value is not well evaluated. Generally, there is an increase of the hormone concentrations in human amniotic fluid. A continous decrease of certain hormones, (e.g., progesterone) remains unexplained.

Characteristic and significant sex differences have been established for amniotic fluid hormone levels (e.g., testosterone, FSH) which are in agreement with the activity of the fetal endocrine system in utero.

With the advent of more extensive use of amniocentesis for prenatal diagnosis and evaluation of fetal lung maturation it was demonstrated that amniotic fluid hormone concentrations can aid in the diagnosis of fetal sex, enzyme defects of fetal organs (e.g., adrenal) and the placenta (e.g., sulfatase deficiency), and the stage of maturation of fetal organs (e.g., lung). With the quantitation of amniotic fluid insulin levels, better control and regulation of maternal carbohydrate metabolism appear to be possible.

The data indicate that the main source of steroids in human amniotic fluid is fetal urine since there is close similarity of the steroid content of amniotic fluid and newborn urine from a qualitative and quantitative point of view. Furthermore, it was shown that the amniotic membranes actively metabolize steroids or secrete hormones (e.g., prolactin), influence the transfer of hormones across the membranes, and might also participate in the initiation of labor.

Hormone uptake by the fetus from the amniotic fluid by deglutition, aspiration, and skin absorption has led to attempts to treat the fetus in utero via amniotic fluid (e.g., fetal adrenal hyperplasia, fetal hypothyroidism).

This review should serve not only to summarize the present knowledge, but also to delineate areas of insufficient knowledge and possibilities for future research.

Acknowledgments

My gratitude is expressed to my teachers in gynecologic endocrinology and biochemistry W. L. Herrmann, P. C. MacDonald, and P. K. Siiteri. The author is indebted to Mrs. Ruth Beeh for her very much appreciated secretarial work. Part of my own studies have been supported by the Ford Foundation, Stiftung Volkswagenwerk, and Deutsche Forschungsgemeinschaft.

References

1. Ostergard DR (1970) The physiology and clinical importance of amniotic fluid. A review. Obstet Gynecol Surv 25:297-319
2. Diczfalusy E (1964) Endocrine functions of the human fetoplacental unit. Fed Proc 23:791–798
3. Diczfalusy E (1969) Steroid metabolism in the human fetoplacental unit. Acta Endocrinol (Copenh) 61:649–664
4. Wynn RM (1974) Development and morphology of the amnion. In: Natelson S, Scommegna A, Epstein MB (eds) Amniotic fluid. Wiley & Sons, New York, pp 3-22
5. Saunders P, Rhodes P (1973) The origin and circulation of amniotic fluid. In: Fairweather DVI, Eskes TKAB (eds) Amniotic fluid. Excerpta Medica, Amsterdam, pp 1-18
6. Bourne GL (1970) The microscopic anatomy of the human amnion and chorion. Am J Obstet Gynecol 79:1070–1073
7. Ahlfeld F (1911) Zwanzig Betrachtungen über die Herkunft des Fruchtwassers. Z Geburtshilfe Gynaekol 69:91–116
8. Jantzen K (1968) Physiologie und Pathologie des Fruchtwassers. Entstehung und Resorption. Gynäk. Rdsch. 5:81-96
9. Seeds AE (1965) Water metabolism of the fetus. Am J Obstet Gynecol 92:727-745
10. Lind T, Cheyne CA (1969) Biochemical and cytological changes in liquor amnii with advancing gestation. J Obstet Gynaecol Br Commonw 76:673–683
11. Behrman RE, Paper JT, Lannoy CW de (1967) Placental growth and the formation of amniotic fluid. Nature 214:678–680
12. Abramovich DR (1973) The volume of amniotic fluid and factors affecting or regulating this. In: Fairweather DVI, Eskes TKA (eds) Amniotic fluid. Excerpta Medica, Amsterdam pp 29–51
13. Koffe S, Godmilow L, Walker BA, Hirschhorn K (1977) Prenatal diagnosis of bilateral renal agenesis. Obstet Gynecol 49:478–480
14. Free AH, Free HM (1974) Laboratory interrelations of amniotic fluid and urine. In: Natelson S, Scommegna, A, Epstein MB (eds) Amniotic fluid. Wiley & Sons, New York, pp 37–46

14a. Anderer M, Schindler AE, Liebich HM (1975) Creatinine, urea and uric acid in amniotic fluid, maternal and umbilical cord blood at delivery. Arch Gynaekol 220:65-72

15. Friedberg V (1955) Untersuchungen über die fetale Urinbildung. Gynaecologia 140:34–45
16. Plentl AA (1960) Formation and circulation of amniotic fluid. Clin Obstet Gynecol 9:427–439
17. Wladimonoff JW, Campbell S (1974) Fetal urine production rates in normal and complicated pregnancies. Lancet I:151–154
18. Abramovich DR, Garden A, Jandial L, Page KR (1979) Fetal swallowing and voiding in relation to hydramnios. Obstet Gynecol 54:15-20
19. Jirasek JE, Capkova A (1969) Concentration of total reducing substances in bladder urine of human midpregnancy fetus after glucose infusion to the mother. Obstet Gynecol 33:805–806
20. Prakasch A, Chalmers JA, Onojobi OIA, Hendersen RJ, Cummings P (1970) Transfer of limocylline and cephalorodine from mother to fetus—a comparative study. J Obstet Gynaecol Br Commonw 77:247–252
21. Bor NM (1964) Circulation of amniotic fluid and its mediating organs. Turk J Pediatr 6:48-53
22. Pitkin RM, Reynolds WA, Berchell RC (1968) Fetal contribution to amniotic fluid. Am J Obstet Gynecol 100:834–838
23. Biggs JS (1970) Production rate and sources of amniotic fluid at term. J Obstet Gynaecol Br Commonw 77:326–332
24. Pritchard JA (1965) Deglutition by normal and anencephalic fetuses. Obstet Gynecol 25: 289-297
25. Pritchard JA (1966) Fetal swallowing and amniotic fluid volume. Obstet Gynecol 28:606–610

26. Grimes LD, Cassadey G (1970) Fetal gastrointestinal obstruction. Am J Obstet Gynecol 106:1196–1200
27. Duenhoelter JH, Pritchard JA (1973) Human fetal respiration. Obstet Gynecol 42:746–750
28. Duenhoelter JH, Pritchard JA (1976) Fetal respiration. Quantitative measurements of amniotic fluid inspired near term by human rhesus fetuses. Am J Obstet Gynecol 125:306–309
29. Harbert GM, Brahme RJ, McGaughey H-S, Thorton WN (1968) Feto-maternal water exchange. Obstet Gynecol 32:232–240
30. Bailey P, Blake M, Younger B, Hinkley C, Cassady G (1976) Amniotic fluid osmolarity in pregnancies complicated by diabetes. Am J Obstet Gynecol 124:257–262
31. Ambramovich DR, Page KR, Jandial L (1976) Bulk flows through human fetal membranes. Gynecol Invest 7:157–164
32. Clements JA, Reyes FI, Winter JDS, Faiman C (1977) Studies on human sexual development. IV. Fetal pituitary and serum and amniotic fluid concentrations of prolactin. J Clin Endocrinol Metab 44:408–413
33. Leontic EA, Andreasson B, Smith B, Tyson JE (1977) Further evidence for the specificity of amniotic osmoregulation by prolactin. Gynecol Invest 8:42
34. Schindler AE, Friedrich E, Barth R, Sparke H, Wuchter J (1974) Steroid profiles in amniotic fluid, cord plasma and newborn urine. In: Schoeller R (ed) Hormonal investigation in pregnancy. Sepe, Paris, pp 603–614
35. Gitling D, Kumate J, Morales C, Noriega L, Arevalo N (1972) The turnover of amniotic fluid protein in the human conceptus. Am J Obstet Gynecol 113:682–645
35a. Seeds AE (1980) Current concepts of amniotic fluid dynamics. Am J Obstet Gynecol 138:575–586
36. Diczfalusy E, Tillinger K-G, Wiqvist N, Levitz M, Condon MS, Dancis J (1963) Disposition of intra-amniotically administered estriol-16-C_1^4 and estrone-16-C^{14} sulfate in women. J Clin Endocrinol Metab 23:503–509
37. Goebelsmann U, Wiqvist N, Diczfalusy E, Levitz M, Condon GP, Dancis J (1966) Fate of intraamniotically administered estriol-15-^{3}H-sulfate and estriol-16-^{14}C-16-glucosideronade in pregnant women at midterm. Acta Endocrinol (Copenh) 52:550–564
38. Katz SR, Dancis J, Levitz M (1965) Relative transfer of estriol and its conjugates across the fetal membranes in vitro. Endocrinology 76:722–727
39. Levitz M (1966) Conjugation and transfer of feto-placental steroid hormones. J Clin Endocrinol Metab 26:773–777
40. Milewich L, Gant NF, Schwarz BE, Prough RA, Chen GT, Athney B, MacDonald PC (1977) Initiation of human parturition. VI. Identification and quantitation of progesterone metabolites produced by components of human fetal membranes. J Clin Endocrinol Metab 45:400–411
41. Milewich L, Gant NF, Schwarz BE, Chen GT, MacDonald PC (1977) Initiation of human parturition. VIII. Metabolism of progesterone by fetal membranes of early and late human gestation. Obstet Gynecol 55:45–48
42. Sulcova J, Jirasek JE, Starka L (1977) The conversion of Δ^5-steroids to testosterone in human amniotic epithelium in vitro. Endokrinologie 70:6–12
43. Sulcova J, Jirasek JE, Starka L (1974) 17β-Hydroxysteroid dehydrogenase activity in human amniotic epithelium. Endokrinologie 63:249–253
44. Sulcova J, Jirasek JE, Carlstedt-Duke J, Starka L (1976) 7-Hydroxylation of dehydroepiandrosterone in human amniotic epithelium. J Steroid Biochem 7:101–104
45. Sulcova J, Capkova A, Jirasek JE, Starka L (1968) 7-Hydroxylation of dehydroepiandrosterone in human foetal liver, adrenals and chorion in vitro. Acta Endocrinol (Copenh) 59: 1–9
46. Tseng L, Stolee S, Gurpide E (1972) In vitro measurements in human placenta and fetal membranes of rates of entry, metabolism and release of steroids. Endocrinology 90:405–414
47. Lopez-Bernal A, Craft I (1979) In vitro cortico-steroid conversion by the human placenta, fetal membranes and decidua in early and late gestation. Br J Obstet Gynaecol 86:387
48. Riddick DH, Kusmik WF (1977) Decidua: A possible source of amniotic fluid prolactin. Am J Obstet Gynecol 127:187–190
49. Walsh SW, Meyer RK, Wolf RC, Friesen HG (1977) Corpus luteum and fetoplacental functions in monkeys hypophysectomized during late pregnancy. Endocrinology 100:845–850
50. Golander A, Hurley T, Barrett J, Hizi A, Handwerger S (1978) Prolactin synthesis by human

chorion-decidual tissue: A possible source of prolactin in the amniotic fluid. Science 20:311-313

51. Healy DL, Kimpton WG, Müller HK, Burger HG (1979) The synthesis of immunoreactive prolactin by decidua-chorion. Br J Obstet Gynaecol 86:307-313
52. Biguzzi M, Pollicino G, Nordi E, Petrucci F, Ronga R, Scarselli GF (1979) Prolactin from human decidua: Specific production and biological activity (abstr). In: Abstract book Serono Symposia Human placenta: Proteins and hormones, Siena 1979, p 62

52a. Riddick DH, Luciano AE, Kusmik WF, Maslar IA (1979) Evidence for a nonpituitary source of amniotic fluid prolactin. Fertil Steril 31:35-39

53. Miettinen TA, Luukkainen T (1968) Gas-liquid chromatography and mass spectrometric studies on steroids in vernix caseosa, amniotic fluid and meconium. Acta Chem Scand [B] 22:2603-2612
54. Wysocki SJ, Hähnel R, Millward MJ, Jenkins DT (1979) Amniotic fluid squalene and fetal maturity. Br J Obstet Gynaecol 86:854-860
55. Singh EJ, Zuspan FP (1973) Amniotic fluid lipids in normal human pregnancy. Am J Obstet Gynecol 117:919-925
56. Nicholas HJ, Schrepper R, Spanos WM, Hunter CA (1963) Steroid relationships confirmed. On the steroid content of amniotic fluid. J Kans Med Soc 64:299-302
57. Schindler AE, Siiteri PK (1968) Isolation and quantitation of steroids from normal human amniotic fluid. J Clin Endocrinol Metab 28:1189-1198
58. Belisle S, Fencl M de M, Ostathanondh R, Tulchinsky D (1978) Sources of 17α-hydroxypregnenolone and its sulfate in human pregnancy. J Clin Endocrinol Metab 46:721-728
59. Luukkainen T, Siegel A, Vihko R (1970) Neutral steroid sulfates in amniotic fluid. J Endrocrinol 40:391-399
60. Jänne O, Vihko R (1970) Presence of 21-hydroxylated neutral steroid disulfates in term amniotic fluid. J Steroid Biochem 1:279-285
61. Zander J, Münstermann A-M (1956) Progesteron im menschlichen Blut und Geweben. III. Progesteron in der Plazenta, in der Uterusschleimhaut und im Fruchtwasser. Klin Wochenschr 34:944-953
62. Friedrich E, Siekmann L, Schindler AE (1975) Identification and quantitation of 16α-hydroxyprogesterone in human amniotic fluid. Clin Chim Acta 56:127-130
63. Frasier SD, Thormegroft IH, Weiss BA, Horton R (1975) Elevated amniotic fluid concentrations of 17α-hydroxyprogesterone in congenital adrenal hyperplasia. J Pediatr 86:310-311
64. Hoet JP, Osinsky PA (1954) Analyses chromatographiques des corticoides extraires du liquide amniotique d'une femme diabétique. Experientia 11:468
65. Baird CW, Bush IE (1960) Cortisol and corticosterone content of amniotic fluid from diabetic and nondiabetic women. Acta Endocrinol (Copenh) 34:97-104
66. Schweitzer M, Klein GP, Giroud CJP (1971) Characterization of 17-deoxy- and 17-hydroxycorticoids in human liquor amnii. J Clin Endocrinol Metab 33:605-611
67. Schweitzer M, Giroud CJP (1971) A comparison of the pattern of steroid glucuronides and sulfates in maternal plasma, umbilical cord plasma and amniotic fluid. J Clin Endocrinol Metab 33:793-798
68. Lambert M, Pennington GW (1973) 6β-Hydroxycortisol in liquor amnii. Nature 197:391-392
69. Lambert M, Pennington GW (1964) Isolation and identification of the 20β-hydroxy derivatives of 6β-hydroxycortisol and 6β-hydroxycorticosterone in liquor amnii. Nature 203:656
70. Pettit BR, Fry DE (1978) Corticosteroids in amniotic fluid and their relationship of fetal lung maturation. J Steroid Biochem 9:1245-1249

70a. Blankstein J, Fujieda K, Reyes FI, Faiman C, Winter JSD (1980) Cortisol, 11-desoxycortisol, and 21-desoxycortisol concentrations in amniotic fluid during pregnancy. Am J Obstet Gynec 137:781-784

70b. Pollack MS, Maurer D, Levine LS, New MI, Pang S, Duchon MA, Owens RP, Merkatz IR, Nitowsky HM, Sachs G, Dupont B (1979) HLA typing of amniotic cells: The prenatal diagnosis of congenital adrenal hyperplasia (21-OH-deficiency type). Transplant Proc 11:1726-1728

71. Aderjan R, Rauh W, Vescei P, Lorenz U, Rüttgers H (1977) Determination of cortisol, tetrahydrocortisol, tetrahydrocortisone, corticosterone and aldosterone in human amniotic fluid. J Steroid Biochem 8:525-528

71a. Blankstein J, Fujieda K, Reyens FI, Faiman C, Winter JSD (1980) Aldosterone and corticosterone in amniotic fluid during various stages of pragnancy. Steroids 36:161-166

72. Peltonen JI, Laatikainen TJ (1975) Steroid glucuronides in amniotic fluid at term. J Steroid Biochem 6:101-105
73. Peltonen JI, Laatikainen TJ, Hesso A (1979) Determination of conjugated steroids in amniotic fluid. J Steroid Biochem 10:499-503
74. Abdine FH, Ghalloungul P, Rili el MS (1954) Über die Zusammensetzung der Amnionflüssigkeit. Hoppe Seylers Z Physiol Chem 296:44-55
75. Klopper AI, MacNaughton MC (1959) The identification of pregnandiol in liquor amnii bile and faeces. J Endocrinol 18:319-325
76. Huhtaniemi I, Vihko R (1970) Quantitation of neutral steroid sulfates in the amniotic fluid of early and mid-pregnancy. Ann Med Exp Biol Fenn 48:188-190
77. Jeffcoate TNA, Fliegner JRH, Russell SH, Davis JC, Wade AP (1965) Diagnosis of the adrenogenital syndrome before birth. Lancet II: 553-555
78. Holzmann K, Wittenbacher G, Mickan H (1974) Pregnanetriol im Fruchtwasser Geburtshilfe Frauenheilkd 34:364-368
79. Rösler A, Leiberman E, Rosenman A, Ben-Uzilio R, Weidenfeld J (1979) Prenatal diagnosis of 11β-hydroxylase deficiency congenital adrenal hyperplasia. J Clin Endocrinol Metab 49:546-551
80. Patti AE, Stein AE (1964) Steroid analysis by gas liquid chromatography. Thomas, Springfield, p 61
81. Siegel AL, Adlercreutz H, Luukkainen T (1969) Gas chromatographic and mass spectrometric identification of neutral and phenolic steroids in amniotic fluid. Ann Med Exp Biol Fenn 47:22-32
82. Tayler NF, Shackleton CHL (1979) Gas chromatographic steroid analysis for diagnosis of placental sulfatase deficiency: A study of nine patients. J Clin Endocrinol Metab 49:78-86
83. Young PE, Judd HL, Robinson JD, Ines OW, Yen SSC (1976) Sex differences of amniotic fluid androgens and estrogens at mid gestation. Gynecol Invest 7:28
84. Vihko R, Hammond GL, Herva R, Tuimula R, Kauppila A (1974) Fetal sex determination by amniotic fluid steroid measurements. J Clin Chem Clin Biochem 15:194
85. Wu CH, Mennuti M, Mikhail G (1977) Free and protein bound hormones in amniotic fluid. Gynecol Invest 8:90-91
86. Mennuti MT, Wu CH, Mellman WJ, Mikhail G (1977) Amniotic fluid testosterone and follicle stimulating hormone levels as indication of fetal sex during mid-pregnancy. Am J Med Genet 1:211-216
87. Nagamani M, McDonough PG, Ellegood JO, Manesh VB (1979) Maternal and amniotic fluid steroid throughout human pregnancy. Am J Obstet Gynecol 134:674-680
88. Saez JM, Bertrand J (1977) Androgen studies in the feto-placental unit. Excerpta Med Int Congr Ser 183:132-141
89. Gandy HM (1971) Androgens. In: Fuchs F, Klopper A (eds) Endocrinology of pregnancy. Harper & Row, New York, pp 101-154
90. Stahl F, Poppe I, Stolzer R, Bindseil R, Dörner G (1972) Testosteronbestimmungen im Plasma und Fruchtwasser mit Hilfe einer kompetitiven Protein-Bindungsmethode. Endokrinologie 60:322-328
91. Dörner G, Stahl F, Rohde W, Halla H, Rössner P, Gruber D, Herter U (1973) Radioimmunologische Bestimmung des Testosterongehalts im Fruchtwasser männlicher und weiblicher Foeten. Endokrinologie 61:317-320
92. Giles HR, Lox D, Heine MW, Christian CD (1974) Intrauterine fetal sex determinations by radioimmunoassay of amniotic fluid testosterone. Gynecol Invest 5:317-323
93. Judd HL, Robinson JD, Young PE, Jones OW (1976) Amniotic fluid testosterone levels in midpregnancy. Obstet Gynecol 48:690-692
94. Belisle S, Fencl M de M, Tulchinsky D (1977) Amniotic fluid testosterone and follicle-stimulating hormone in the determination of fetal sex. Am J Obstet Gynecol 128:514-519
95. Dörner G, Stahl F, Rohde W, Göretzlehner G, Witkowski R, Saffert H (1977) Sex-specific testosterone and FSH concentrations in amniotic fluid of mid-pregnancy. Endokrinologie 70:86-88
96. Künzig HJ, Mayer U, Schmitz-Roeckerath B, Broer KH (1977) Influence of fetal sex on the concentration of amniotic fluid testosterone: Antinatal sex determination? Arch Gynaekol 223:75-84

97. Zondek T, Mansfield MD, Zondek LH (1977) Amniotic fluid testosterone and fetal sex determination in the first half of pregnancy. Br J Obstet Gynaecol 84:714–716
98. Dawood MY, Saxena BB (1977) Testosterone and dihydrotestosterone in maternal and cord blood and in amniotic fluid. Am J Obstet Gynecol 129:37–42
99. Warne GL, Faiman C, Reyes FI, Winter JSD (1977) Studies on human sexual development. V. Concentrations of testosterone, 17-hydroxyprogesterone in human amniotic fluid throughout gestation. J Clin Endocrinol Metab 44:934–938
100. Ketupanya A, Wiest WG (1978) Amniotic fluid testosterone concentration as an index of fetal sex. Pediatr Res 12:708–710
101. Pirani BBK, Pairandeau N, Dorant A, Wong PY, Gardner HA (1977) Amniotic fluid testosterone in the prenatal determination of fetal sex. Am J Obstet Gynecol 109:518–520
102. Distler W, Boniver-Ollmann U, Claussen U, Tigges J, Terinde R (1979) Radioimmunologische Bestimmung von Testosteron mit und ohne Chromatographie des Fruchtwassers zur pränatalen Geschlechtsdiagnose. Arch Gynecol 227:7-12
103. Luukkainen T, Michie EA, Vihko R (1971) Disulfates of neutral steroids in the amniotic fluid from anencephalic pregnancies. J Endocrinol 51:109–115
104. Diczfalusy E (1953) Chorionic gonadotropin and estrogens in the human placenta. Acta Endocrinol [Suppl 12] 12:141–143
105. Diczfalusy E, Magnusson A-M (1958) Tissue concentration of estrone, estradiol-17β and estriol in the human fetus. Acta Endocrinol 28:169-185
106. Wodrig W, Göretzlehner G (1964) Untersuchungen über den Östrogenspiegel im Blutserum und Fruchtwasser bei Diabetes mellitus und Schwangerschaft. Z Geburtshilfe Gynaekol 182:89–94
107. Michie EA (1966) Estrogen levels in urine and amniotic fluid in pregnancy with live anencephalic fetus and the effect of intraamniotic injection of sodium dehydroepiandrosterone sulfate on these levels. Acta Endocrinol (Copenh) 51: 535-542
108. Drafta D, Cristoveanu A, Tache A, Stroe E, Ciocirdia C, Roman L (1972) Steroids in the amniotic fluid. Rev Roum Endocrinol 9:197–206
109. Adlercreutz H, Luukkainen T (1970) Identification and determination of estrogens in various biological materials in pregnancy. Ann Clin Res 2:365-380
110. Schindler AE, Herrmann WL (1966) Estriol in pregnancy urine and amniotic fluid. Am J Obstet Gynecol 95:301-307
111. Emara SH, El-Hawary MF, Abdel Karim HA, El-Heneidy FM (1976) Total lipids, cholesterol, phospholipids and inorganic phosphorus in the amniotic fluid of premature infants. S Afr Med J 50:1792-1794
112. Giraud JR, Muraine J, Touron M, Reiss D, Gombert J (1972) Composition du liquide amniotique en fin de grossesse 2. – Première résultats sur 230 grossesses, concernant le phosphore, le calcium, le cholesterol, le glucose, le sodium, le potassium, le chlore et les bicarbonates. J Gynecol Obstet Biol Reprod (Paris) 1:795–804
113. Anton W, Hofmann D, Fischer J (1973) Cholesterinspiegel und Reststickstoff im menschlichen Fruchtwasser bei normaler und gestörter Gravidität. Zentralbl Gynaekol 95:1844–1850
114. Weisberg HF (1974) Clinical chemical analysis of sixty-two amniotic fluids from women in early pregnancy. In: Natelson S, Scomegna A, Epstein MB (eds) Amniotic fluid. Wiley & Sons, New York, pp 47-71
115. Schindler AE, Anderer HM, Liebich HM (1978) Cholesterol in amniotic fluid, maternal and umbilical cord blood. Arch Gynaecol 226:289-296
116. Owen VMJ, Ho FK, Mazzuchin A, Doran TA, Liedgren S, Porter CJ (1976) Cholesterol in amniotic fluid, determined by gas chromatography. Clin Chem 22:224-226
117. Fennefrohn B (1972) Fruchtwasseruntersuchungen in den letzten Schwangerschaftswochen. Z Geburtshilfe Perinatol 176:233-241
118. Bonsnes RW (1966) Composition of amniotic fluid. Clin Obstet Gynecol 9:440–448
119. Wolf PL, Bloch D, Tsudaka T (1970) Biochemical profile of amniotic fluid, to assess fetal maturity. Clin Chem 16:843-844
120. Huchinson DL (1967) Amniotic fluid. In: Marcus SL, Marcus CC Advances in obstetrics and gynecology. (eds) Williams & Wilkins, Baltimore, pp 125–130
121. Milunsky A, Tulchinsky D (1977) Prenatal diagnosis of congenital adrenal hyperplasia due to 21-hydroxylase deficiency. Pediatrics 59:768–769

122. Harbert GM, McGaughey HS, Scoggin WA, Thorton WN (1964) Concentration of progesterone in newborn and maternal circulations at delivery. Obstet Gynecol 23:413-426
123. Lurie AO, Reid DE, Villee CA (1966) The role of the fetus and placenta in maintenance of plasma progesterone. Am J Obstet Gynecol 96:670-675
124. Wiest WG (1967) Estimation of progesterone in biological tissues and fluids from pregnant women by double isotope derivative. Steroids 10:279-290
125. Younglai EV, Effer SB, Pelletier C (1971) Amniotic fluid progestins and estrogens in relation to length of gestation. Am J Obstet Gynecol 111:833-839
126. Johansson EDB, Jonasson L-E (1971) Progesterone levels in amniotic fluid and plasma from women. I. Levels during normal pregnancy. Acta Obstet Gynecol Scand 50:339-343
127. Younglai EV, Pelletier C (1972) A competitive protein-binding method for the measurement of progesterone in human amniotic fluid. J Steroid Biochem 3:919-924
128. Koren Z, Schulman H, Lev-Gur M, Gatz M, Thysen B, Bloch E (1976) Progesterone levels in amniotic fluid and maternal plasma in prostaglandin $F_{2\alpha}$-induced midtrimester abortion. Obstet Gynecol 48:472-474
129. Göser R, Meierl W, Schindler AE (to be published) Radioimmunologische Bestimmungen von Östron, Östradiol, Östriol, Progesteron, Cortisol und Prolaktin aus dem Fruchtwasser von normalen und pathologischen Schwangerschaften
130. Pulkkinen MO, Enkola K (1972) The progesterone gradient of the human fetal membranes. Int J Obstet Gynaecol 10:93-94
131. Ylikorkala O, Dawood MY, Kauppila A, Tuimala R (1978) Effect of maternal dexamethasone therapy on the levels of estrogens, progesterone and chorionic gonadotrophin in amniotic fluid and maternal serum. Br J Obstet Gynaecol 85:334-337
132. Jonasson L-E, Johansson EDB (1971) Progesterone levels in amniotic fluid and plasma from women. II. Levels during pregnancies complicated by Rh-isoimmunization or hepatosis gravidarum. Acta Obstet Gynecol Scand 50:345-350
133. Schindler AE, Keller E (1973) Grundlagen des Steroidstoffwechsels bei Schwangerschaften mit Rh-Inkompatibilität. Z Geburtshilfe Perinatol 177:305-314
134. Varma K, Heine MW, Haller WS, Row AD, Railsback K, Varma SK (1979) Ratio of amniotic fluid cortisol and maternal cortisol (AFC/MSC) as an index of fetal lung maturity. Acta Obstet Gynecol Scand 58:439-442
135. Ohrlander S, Gennser G, Batra S, Lebech P (1977) Effect of betamethasone administration on estrone, estradiol-17β and progesterone in maternal plasma and amniotic fluid. Obstet Gynecol 49:148-153
136. Tulchinsky D, Simmer HH (1972) Sources of plasma 17α-hydroxyprogesterone in human pregnancy. J Clin Endocrinol Metab 35:799-808
137. Hagemenas FC, Kittinger WC (1973) The influence of fetal sex in the levels of plasma progesterone in the human fetus. J Clin Endocrinol Metab 36:389
138. Nagamani M, McDonough PG, Ellgood JO, Mahesh VB (1978) Maternal and amniotic fluid 17α-hydroxyprogesterone levels during pregnancy: Diagnosis of congenital adrenal hyperplasia in utero. Am J Obstet Gynecol 130:791-794
139. Cope CL, Hurlock B, Sewell C (1955) The distribution of adrenal corticol hormone in some body fluids. Clin Sci 14:25-36
140. Pokoly TB (1973) The role of cortisol in human parturition. Am J Obstet Gynecol 117:549-553
141. Jolivet A (1974) Cortisol in amniotic fluid and human parturition. J Steroid Biochem 5:367
142. Sybulski S, Maughan GB (1975) A rapid method for the measurement of estradiol and hydrocortisone levels in maternal and fetal blood and amniotic fluid. J Obstet Gynecol 121:32-36
143. Fencl M de M, Tulchinsky D (1975) Total cortisol in amniotic fluid and fetal lung maturation. N Engl J Med 292:133-136
144. Murphy BEP, Patrick J, Denton RL (1975) Cortisol in amniotic fluid during human gestation. J Clin Endocrinol Metab 40:164-167
145. Häffele R, Eichelberg G, König A (1975) Oestrogene und Cortisol im Fruchtwasser bei normal und pathologisch verlaufender Schwangerschaft. Z Geburtshilfe Perinatol 179:437-440
146. Murphy BEP (1975) Non-chromatographic radiotransinassay for cortisol: Application to human adult serum, umbilical cord serum, and amniotic fluid. J Clin Endocrinol Metab 40:1050-1057

147. Sivakumaran F, Duncan ML, Effer SB, Younglai EV (1975) Relationship between cortisol and lecithin/sphingomyelin ratios in human amniotic fluid. Am J Obstet Gynecol 122:291-294
148. Ohrlander SAV, Gennser GM, Grennert L (1975) Impact of betamethasone load given to pregnant women on endocrine balance of fetoplacental unit. Am J Obstet Gynecol 123:228-236
149. Tuimala R, Kuappila A, Rönnberg L, Jouppila R, Haapilahti J (1976) The effect of labour on ACTH and cortisol levels in amniotic fluid and maternal blood. Br J Obstet Gynaecol 83:707-710
150. Tan SY, Gewolb IH, Hobbins JC (1976) Unconjugated cortisol in human amniotic fluid: Relationship to lecithin/sphingomyelin ratio. J Clin Endocrinol Metab 43:412-418
151. Onishi K, Matsunaga T, Yamaje K, Miyuzo AG, Inagaki H (1974) Comparison of steroid patterns in maternal and fetal sera and in the amniotic fluid expressed in high speed liquid chromatography and evaluation of their changes after delivery. Clin Endocrinol (Tokyo) 24:303-313
152. Smith BT, Worthington D, Malony AHA (1977) Fetal lung maturation. III. The amniotic fluid cortisol/cortisone ratio in preterm human delivery and the risk of respiratory distress syndrome. Obstet Gynecol 49:527-531
153. Sharp-Cageorge SM, Blocher BM, Gordon ER, Murphy BEP (1977) Amniotic fluid cortisol and human fetal lung maturation. N Engl J Med 296:89-92
154. Koren Z, Leo-Gur M, Gatz M, Randolph G, Thysen B, Bloch E, Schulman H (1977) Cortisol levels in amniotic fluid in prostaglandin $F_{2\alpha}$-induced midtrimester abortion. Am J Obstet Gynecol 127:639-642
155. Sybulski S (1977) Effect of antepartum betamethasone treatment on cortisol levels in cord plasma, amniotic fluid and the neonate. Am J Obstet Gynecol 127:871-874
156. Mackenzie IZ, Pooley G, Challis JRG (1977) Changes in the concentration of cortisol in amniotic fluid after intra-amniotic prostaglandin for midtrimester abortion. Br J Obstet Gynaecol 84:608-612
157. Johnson B, Hensleigh PA (1977) Surfactant test and amniotic fluid cortisol. Am J Obstet Gynecol 129:105-107
158. Peltonen J, Vinikka L, Laatikainen T (1977) Amniotic fluid cortisol during gestation and its relation to fetal lung maturation. J Steroid Biochem 8:1159-1163
159. Björkhem J, Lautto O, Lunell N-O, Pshera H (1978) Total and free cortisol in amniotic fluid during late pregnancy. Br J Obstet Gynaecol 85:446-450
160. Herbst J, Wickens EJ, Quakarnack K, Dame WR, Nieschlag E (1978) Cortisol im Fruchtwasser und im mütterlichen Blut – ein Parameter zur Bestimmung der fetalen Lungenreife. Z Geburtshilfe Perinatol 132:212-218
161. Doran TA, Ford JA, Allen LC, Wong PY, Benzie RJ (1979) Amniotic fluid lecithin/sphingomyelin ratio, palmitic acid/ stearic acid ratio, total cortisol, creatinine, and percentage of lipid positive cells in assessment of fetal maturity and fetal pulmonary maturity: A comparison. Am J Obstet Gynecol 133:302-307
162. Gennser G, Ohrlander S, Enneroth P (1976) Cortisol in amniotic fluid and cord blood in relation to prenatal betamethasone load and delivery. Am J Obstet Gynecol 124:43–50
163. Gewolb IH, Hobbins JC, Tan SY (1977) Amniotic fluid cortisol in high-risk human pregnancies. Obstet Gynecol 49:466-470
164. Goldkrant JW (1978) Unconjugated estriol and cortisol in maternal and cord serum and amniotic fluid in normal and abnormal pregnancy. Obstet Gynecol 52:264-271
165. Jolivet A, Gautray J-P (1977) Variations des stéroides non conjugués dans le liquide amniotique au cours des dernières semaines de la grossesse. CR Acad Sci [D] (Paris) 284:1127–1129
166. Bruzy JE, Grenshaw MC, Brumley GW (1978) Amniotic fluid cortisol in normal and diabetic pregnant women and its relation to respiratory disease in the neonate. Am J Obstet Gynecol 132:567-570
167. Liggins GC, Fairclough RJ, Grieves SA, Kendall JC, Knox BS (1973) The mechanism of initiation of parturition in the ewe. Recent Prog Horm Res 29:111–149
168. Liggins GC, Howie RN (1972) A controlled trial for ante-partum glucocorticoid treatment for prevention of the respiratory distress syndrome in premature infants. Pediatrics 50:515-525
169. Murphy BEP (1974) Cortisol and cortisone levels in cord blood at delivery of infants with and without respiratory distress syndrome. Am J Obstet Gynecol 119:1112
170. Kuss E (1976) Biochemie und präpartale Diagnostik der Lungenreife. J Clin Chem Clin Biochem 14:505-513

171. Hallmann M, Gluck L (1977) Development of the fetal lung. J Perinat Med 5:3-31
172. Kuwabara Y, Misaki N, Sato K, Jinbo T, Suzuki T (1974) Cortisol and estriol dynamics in the amniotic fluid. Folia Endocrinol 50:621
173. Bauer CR, Stern L, Colle E (1974) Prolonged rupture of the membranes associated with decreased incidence of respiratory distress syndrome. Pediatrics 53:7-12
173a. Cohen W, Fencl M de M, Tulchinsky D (1976) Amniotic fluid cortisol after premature rupture of membranes. J Pediatr 88:1007-1009
174. Bichler A, Geir W (1979) Palmitinsäure im Fruchtwasser bei pathologischen Schwangerschaften. Arch Gynaecol 227:13-27
175. Fencl M de M, Osathanondh R, Tulchinsky D (1967) Plasma cortisol and cortisone in pregnancies with normal and anencephalic fetuses. J Clin Endocrinol Metab 43:80-85
176. Sybulski S, Maighan GB (1976) Cortisol levels in umbilical cord plasma in relation to labor and delivery. Am J Obstet Gynecol 125:236-238
177. Hensleigh PA, Moore WV, Wilson K, Tulchinsky D (1978) Congenital x-linked adrenal hypoplasia. Obstet Gynecol 52:228-232
178. Braunstein GD, Ziel FH, Allen A, Vehlde van de R, Wade ME (1976) Prenatal diagnosis of placental steroid sulfatase deficiency. Am J Obstet Gynecol 126:716-719
179. Bruhashi N, Suzuki M, Fukaya T, Kono H, Tachibana Y, Shinkawa O (1980) Cephalothoracopagus: Case report with endocrine study. Arch Gynaecol 229:161-166
179a. Simmer HH, Frankland M, Greipel M (1975) On the regulation of fetal and maternal 16αOH-dehydroepiandrosterone and its sulfate by cortisol and ACTH in human pregnancy at term. Am J Obstet Gynecol 121:646-652
180. Diedrich K, Stefan M, Krebs D (1978) The effect of betamethasone therapy on the L/S ratio in amniotic fluid. J Perinat Med 6:22-27
181. Lambert M, Pennington GW (1965) The estimation of polar steroids in liquor amnii. J Endocrinol 32:287-293
182. Schumert Z, Rosenmann A, Landau H, Rösler A (1980) 11-Deoxycortisol in amniotic fluid: Prenatal diagnosis of congenital adrenal hyperplasia due to 11β-hydroxylase deficiency. Clin Endocrinol 12:257-260
183. Pennington GW (1965) Adrenogenital syndrome before birth. Lancet II:848-849
184. Schindler AE, Ratanasopa V (1968) Profile of steroids in amniotic fluid of normal and complicated pregnancies. Acta Endocrinol (copenh) 59:239-248
185. Klopper A, Wilson GR, Shearman RP (1970) A method for the estimation of pregnanediol in amniotic fluid. J Obstet Gynaecol Br Commonw 77:531-535
186. Clarke A, Klopper A (1970) The measurement of pregnanediol sulfate in amniotic fluid. J Endocrinol 46:123-124
187. Woyton J, Sward J, Dzioba A, Gajewski A, Szacki J, Basanowski H (1973) Behaviour of total oestrogen, pregnanediol and creatinine levels in the amniotic fluid in the last weeks of gestation. J Obstet Gynaecol Br Commonw 80:909-911
188. Schindler AE (1972) Steroide im Fruchtwasser. Fortschr. Geburtshilfe Gynaekol 46:1-89
189. Merkatz IR, New MI, Petorson RE, Seaman MP (1969) Prenatal diagnosis of adrenogenital syndrome by amniocentesis. J Pediatr 75:977-982
190. Nichols J (1969) Antenatal diagnosis of adrenocortical hyperplasia. Lancet I:1151-1152
191. Nichols J, Gibson GG (1969) Antenatal diagnosis of the adrenogenital syndrome. Lancet II: 1068-1069
192. Nichols J (1970) Antenatal diagnosis and treatment of the adrenogenital syndrome. Lancet I:83
193. Wade AP, Abramovich DR (1967) The distribution of 17-oxosteroids and 17-hydroxy-corticosteroids in amniotic fluid. Steroids 10:669-686
194. Abramovich DR, Wade AP (1969) Levels and significance of 17-oxosteroids and 17-hydroxycorticosteroids in amniotic fluid throughout pregnancy. J Obstet Gynaecol Br Commonw 76:893-897
195. Gadd RL (1966) The volume of liquor amnii in normal and abnormal pregnancies. J Obstet Gynaecol Br Commonw 73:11-22
196. Dörner G, Stahl F, Baumgarten F (1972) Signifikante Unterschiede im Testosteron- und 11-OHCS-Gehalt des Fruchtwassers zwischen männlichen und weiblichen Föten. Endokrinologie 60:285-288

197. Mukherjee TK, Roth M, Recht L, Meredith N, Sirmans MF, Batts JA (1977) Significance of amniotic fluid corticosteroid levels in human pregnancies. Obstets Gynecol 49:144-147
198. Warne GL, Reyes FL, Faiman C, Winter JSD (1978) Studies on human sexual development. VI. Concentrations of unconjugated dehydroepiandrosterone, estradiol and estriol in amniotic fluid throughout gestation. J Clin Endocrinol Metab 47:1363-1367
199. Robinson JD, Judd HL, Young PE, Jones OW, Yen SSC (1977) Amniotic fluid androgens and estrogens in midgestation. J Clin Endocrinol Metab 45:755-761
200. Dvorák P, Hampl R, Macek M, Chrpova M, Burjankova J, Starka L (1980) Free dehydroepiandrosterone and testosterone in human amniotic fluid and prediction of gonadal sex. Endocrinol Exp (Bratisl) 14:59-66
201. Osathanondh R, Canick J, Ryan KJ, Tulchinsky D (1976) Placental sulfatase deficiency: A case study. J Clin Endocrinol Metab 43:208-214
202. France JT (1969) A placental steroid sulfatase defect in human pregnancy. Master's thesis, University of Auckland
203. Bierbaum U (1976) Steroidkonzentration im Fruchtwasser und mütterlichen Blut bei normaler und pathologischer Schwangerschaft. Med. Dissertation, Universität Homburg
204. Mancuso S, Bellante FP, Angelini A, Marana R (1980) Amniotic 5-androstene-3β, 17α-diol in high risk pregnancy. J Steroid Biochem 12:95-96
205. Menini E, Bellarti U (1970) Estriol and estriol related compounds in amniotic fluid from normal and pathological pregnancies. Ann Obstet Ginecol Med Perinat Special number 101-105
206. Abramovich DR, Wade AP (1969) Transplacental passage of steroids: The presence of corticosteroids in amniotic fluid. J Obstet Gynaecol Br Commonw 76:610-614
207. Reyes FI, Boroditsky RS, Winter JSD, Faiman C (1974) Studies on human sexual development. II. Fetal and maternal serum gonadotropin and sex steroid concentration. J Clin Endocrinol Metab 38:612-617
208. Younglai EV, Lin C-C (1973) Fetal endrogen and human chorionic gonadotropin excretion in relation to genetic sex. Am J Obstet Gynecol 117:291-292
209. Frasier SD, Weiss BA, Horten R (1974) Amniotic fluid testosterone: Implications for the prenatal diagnosis of congenital adrenal hyperplasia. J Pediatr 84:738-741
210. Doran TA, Wong PY, Allen LG, Falk M (1980) Amniotic fluid testosterone and follicle--stimulating hormone assay in the prenatal determination of fetal sex. Am J Obstet Gynecol 136:309-312
210a. Zondek T, Fox J, Zondek LH (1980) Amniotic fluid follicle-stimulation hormone and fetal sex determination in the second trimester of pregnancy. J Obstet Gynaecol 1:12-16
211. Robertson RD, Henniker AJ, Luttrell BM, Saunders DM (1980) The prenatal determination of fetal sex: Amniotic fluid testosterone as preliminary screening test. Eur J Obstet Gynecol Reprod Biol 10:77-81
212. Mizuno M, Lobosky J, Lloyd CW, Kobayashi T, Murasawa Y (1968) Plasma androstenedione and testosterone during pregnancy and in the newborn. J Clin Endocrinol Metab 28:1133-1142
213. Abramovich DR, Rowe P (1973) Fetal plasma testosterone levels at midpregnancy and at term. Relationship to fetal sex. J Endocrinol 56:621-622
214. Berman AM, Kalchman GG, Chattoraj SC, Scomegna A (1968) Relationship of amniotic estriol to maternal urinary estriol. Am J Obstet Gynecol 100:15-23
215. Gillet J-Y, Duperval R, Koller B, Wulff F, Mandel P, Müller P (1971) Le dosage de l'œstriol dans le liquide amniotique: Valeurs normales — intérêt et signification dans les grossesses pathologiques. Gynecol Obstet 70:447-456
215a. Muller P, Dellenbach P, Vors J, Guikovaty JP, Masson D, Lavalleye Ph, Viteux V, Lemmer R, Schick AR (1974) Etude de l'œstriol au cours de la grossesse normale et de ses principales variantes pathologiques dans le liquide amniotique. In: Scholler R (ed) Hormone investigations in human pregnancy. Sepe, Paris, pp 615-643
216. Roy EJ (1972) The concentration of estrogens in maternal and fetal blood obtained at cesarean section and the effect of hospitalisation on maternal blood estrogen levels. J Obstet Gynaecol Br Commonw 69:196-202
217. Aleem FA, Neill DW, Pinkerton JHM (1969) A method for estriol estimation in amniotic fluid and its use in the study of normal and abnormal pregnancy. Steroids 13:651-670

218. Michie EA, Livingstone JR (1969) Estriol concentration in amniotic fluid. Acta Endocrinol (Copenh) 61:329-333
219. Fencl M de M, Alonso C, Alba M (1972) Estriol values in amniotic fluid in the course of normal pregnancy. Am J Obstet Gynecol 113:367-371
220. Jörgensen PI, Frandsen AV, Svenstrup B (1974) Amniotic fluid estriol concentration during the last trimester of pregnancy. I. Normal pregnancy. Acta Obstet Gynecol Scand 53:23-28
221. Touchstone JC, Murawec T, Bolognese RJ (1972) Gas-chromatographic determination of total estriol in amniotic fluid. Clin Chem 38:129-130
222. Klopper A (1972) Estriol in liquor amnii. Am J Obstet Gynecol 112:129-130
223. Schindler AE, Ratanasopa V, Lee TY, Hermann WL (1967) Estriol and RH-isoimmunization: A new approach to the management of severely affected pregnancies. Obstet Gynecol 29:625-631
224. Bolognese RJ, Carson SL, Tochstone JC, Lakoff KM (1971) Correlation of amniotic fluid estriol with fetal age and well-being. Obstet Gynecol 37:437-441
225. Aleem FA, Pinkerton JHM, Neill DW (1969) Clinical significance of the amniotic fluid estriol level. J Obstet Gynaecol Br Commonw 76:200-207
226. Bacigalupo G, Dudenhausen JW, Saling E (1977) Role of assays of total estriol in amniotic fluid for the diagnosis of fetal hypotrophy. J Perinat Med 5:76-83
227. Ryn S, Hoshaku K, Kosaka J, Fujiwara Y (1974) Determination of estriol in the amniotic fluid by amberlite XAD—2. Clin Endocrinol (Tokyo) 22:1091-1094
228. Bacigalupo G, Saling EZ, Dudenhausen JW (1979) Unconjugated and total estriol in human amniotic fluid—changes in the ratios between the two estriol levels with advancing gestation age. J Perinat Med 70:262-269
229. Giraud JR, Muraine J, Gibonin L, Reiss D (1970) Étude de la concentration on estriol du liquide amniotique en function du poids du foetus et du terme de la gestation dans les grossesses normales. Bull Fed Soc Gynecol Obstet Lang Fr 22:281-286
230. Perez-Lopez FR, Roncero MC, Canes E, Davi E, Saltukoglu A (1974) Estriol levels in human amniotic fluid. J Steroid Biochem 5:362
231. Oszczygiel A (1976) Oestrogenspiegel im Fruchtwasser vor der Geburt. Zentralbl Gynaekol 98:725-728
232. Troen P, Nilsson B, Wiqvist N, Diszefalusy E (1961) Pattern of estriol conjugates in human cord blood, amniotic fluid and urine of the newborn. Acta Endocrinol (Copenh) 38:361-384
233. Diczfaluzy E, Lauritzen C (eds) (1961) Oestrogene beim Menschen. Springer, Berlin, p 337
234. Klopper A, Bíggs J (1970) The correlation between urinary estriol excretion and the estriol concentration in liquor amnii. J Endocrinol 48:471-472
235. Goebelsmann U, Work BA (1970) Estriol conjugates in amniotic fluid in normal pregnancies and Rh-isoimmunization. Gynecol Invest 1:222-223
236. Sobrevilla LA, Romero I, Kruger F (1971) Estriol levels of cord blood, maternal venous blood and amniotic fluid at delivery at high altitude. Am J Obstet Gynecol 110:596-597
237. Young BK, Jirku H, Levite M (1972) Estriol conjugates in amniotic fluid at midpregnancy at term. J Clin Endocrinol Metab 35:208-212
238. Sciarra JJ, Tagatz GE, Notation AP, Depp R (1974) Estriol and estetrol in amniotic fluid. Am J Obstet Gynecol 118:626-642
239. Gurpide E, Giebenhain ME, Tseng L, Kelley WG (1971) Radioimmunoassay for estrogens in human pregnancy urine, plasma and amniotic fluid. Am J Obstet Gynecol 109:897-906
240. Jörgensen PI (1974) Amniotic fluid estriol, concentration during the last trimester of pregnancy. II. Perinatal mortality and morbidity. Acta Obstet Gynecol Scand 53:29-36
241. Giraud JR, Muraine J, Gibonin L, Reiss D (1972) Caractères du liquide amniotique en fin de grossesse. 1. Concentration en estriol. J Gynecol Obstet Biol Reprod (Paris)1:309-322
242. Feuillu A, Rio M, Taillanter L, Cormier M (1974) Intérêt du dosage de l'œstriol de la creatinine et de la dermination chromatographique des phospholipides dans le liquide amniotique. Ann Biol Clin (Paris) 32:347-352
243. Biggs JS, Klopper A (1969) The variability of estriol concentration in amniotic fluid. J Obstet Gynaecol Br Commonw 76:999-1002
244. Biggs JS (1969) Estriol in amniotic fluid: The effect of storage, filtration and glucose. J Endocrinol 48:607-608
245. Klopper A, Michie E, Aleem F (1971) The estimation of estriol in amniotic fluid: A comparison of three methods. J Obstet Gynaecol Br Commonw 78:444-447

246. Michie EA, Robertson JG (1971) Amniotic and urinary estriol assays in pregnancies complicated by rhesus isoimmunization. J Obstet Gynaecol Br Commonw 78:34–40
247. Young BK, Jirku H, Slyper AJ, Levitz M, Kelley WG, Yaverbaum S (1974) Estriol conjugates in amniotic fluid of normal and Rh-isoimmunized patients. J Clin Endocrinol Metab 38:842–849
248. Tikkanen MJ, Adlercreutz H (1973) Estriol conjugates in amniotic fluid. Qualitative and quantitative aspects including preliminary studies in Rh-isoimmunization. Acta Endocrinol (Copenh) 73:555–566
249. Hinkley C, O'Neil L, Cassady G (1973) Amniotic fluid creatinine in the Rh-sensitized pregnancy. Am J Obstet Gynecol 117:544–548
250. Heikkila J, Lukkainen T (1971) Urinary excretion of estriol and 15-hydroxyestriol in complicated pregnancies. Am J Obstet Gynecol 110:509–521
251. Tulchinsky D, Frigoletti FD, Ryan JK, Fishman J (1975) Plasma estetrol as an index of fetal well-being. J Clin Endocrinol Metab 40:560–567
252. Notation AE, Tagatz GE (1977) Unconjugated estriol and 15-hydroxyestriol in complicated pregnancies. Am J Obstet Gynecol 128:747–756
253. Murphy BEP (1978) Conjugated glucocorticoids in amniotic fluid and fetal lung maturation. J Clin Endocrinol Metab 47:212–215
254. Murphy BEP, Silverman AY (1979) Comparison of glucocorticoid conjugates with other indices of fetal maturation. Obstet Gynecol 54:35-38
255. Klopper A (1974) Estriol amniotic fluid. In: Persianinow LS, Chervakova TV (eds) Recent progress in obstetrics and gynecology. Excerpta Medica, Amsterdam, pp 162–169
256. Levitz M, Jirku H, Kadner S, Young BK (1975) Estriol conjugates in body fluids in late human pregnancy. J Steroid Biochem 6:663–667
257. Levitz M, Kadner S, Young BK (1976) 16-Sulfates of estriol in body fluids of human pregnancy at term. Steroids 27:287-294
258. Sugar J, Dessy C, Alexander S, Amy J-J, Rodesch F, Schwers J (1980) Estriol-3-glucuronide and E_3-16-glucuronide in amniotic fluid during normal pregnancy. J Clin Endocrinol Metab 50:137-141
259. Klein GP, Chan SK, Giroud CJP (1969) Urinary excretion of 17-hydroxy- and 17-desoxysteroids of the preg-4-ene series by the human newborn. J Clin Endocrinol Metab 29:1448–1455
260. Schindler AE, Friedrich E, Barth R, Sparke H, Wuchter J (1974) Steroid profiles in amniotic fluid, cord plasma and newborn urine. In: Scholler R (ed) Hormonal investigations in human pregnancy. Sepe, Paris, pp 603–613
261. Migeon CJ, Bertrand J, Gemzell CA (1961) The transplacental passage of various steroid hormones in mid-pregnancy. Recent Prog Horm Res 17:207-248
262. Bolte E, Mancuso S, Eriksson G, Wiqvist N, Diczfaluzy E (1964) Studies on the aromatization of neutral steroids in pregnant women. 2. Aromatization of dehydroepiandrostorene and of its sulfate administered simultaneously in to an uterine artery. Acta Endocrinol 45:560
263. Diczfalusy E, Cassmer O, Alonso C, De Miguel M (1961) Estrogen metabolism in the human fetus and newborn. Recent Prog Horm Res 17:147-206
264. Diczfalusy E, Tillinger K-G, Wiqvist N, Levitz M, Condon GP, Dancis J (1963) Disposition of intraamniotically administered estriol-16-C^{14} and estrone-16-C^{14} sulfate by women. J Clin Endocrinol Metab 23:503-509
265. Katz SR, Dancis J, Levitz M (1965) Relative transfer of estriol and its conjugates across the fetal membranes in vitro. Endocrinology 76:723-227
266. Levitz M (1966) Conjugation and transfer of fetal-placental steroid hormones. J Clin Endocrinol Metab 26:773–777
267. Gant NF, Milewich L, Calvert ME, MacDonald PC (1977) Steroid sulfatase activity in human fetal membranes. J Clin Endocrinol Metab 45:965–972
268. Goebelsmann U, Wiqvist N, Diczfalusy S, Levitz M, Condon GP, Dancis J (1966) Fate of intraamniotically administered estriol-16-^{3}H-sulfate and estriol-16-^{14}C-16-glucosiduronate in pregnant women at midterm. Acata Endocrinol (Copenh) 52:555–564
271a. Tanswell AK, Worthington D, Smith BT (1977) Human amniotic membrane corticosteroid 11-oxidoreductase activity. J Clin Endocrinol Metab 45:721–725
271b. Tanswell AK, Smith BT (1978) The relationship of amniotic membrane 11-oxido-reductase activity to lung maturation in the human fetus. Pediatr Res 12:957-960

269. Barnes AC, Kumar D, Goodno JA (1962) Studies in human myometrium during pregnancy. V. Myometrial tissue progesterone analysis by gas-liquid-phase chromatography. Am J Obstet Gynecol 84:1207
270. Runnebaum B, Zander J (1971) Progesterone and 20α-dihydroxyprogesterone in human pregnancy. Acta Endocrinol [Suppl] (Copenh) 150:5
271. Murphy BEP (1977) Chorionic membrane as an extra-adrenal source of fetal cortisol in human amniotic fluid. Nature 266:179–181
272. Schwarz BE, Milewich L, Gant NF, Porter JC, Johnston JM, MacDonald PC (1977) Progesterone binding and metabolism in human fetal membranes. Ann NY Acad Sci 286:304–312
273. Gibb W, Lavoie J-C, Roux J (1980) In vitro conversion of pregnenolone to progesterone by term human fetal membranes. Am J Obstet Gynecol 136:631–634
274. Milewich L, Gant NF, Schwarz BE, Chen GT, MacDonald PC (1979) Initiation of human parturition. VII. Partial characterization of progesterone metabolizing enzymes of human amnion and chorion leave J Steroid Biochem 11:1577-1582
275. Beling CG, Cederqvist LL (1978) Progesterone metabolism in cultured amniotic fluid cells. Int J Gynaecol Obstet 15:317-321
276. Siiteri PK, Wilson JD (1974) Testosterone formation and metabolism during male sexual differentiation in the human embryo. J Clin Endocrinol Metab 38:113–125
277. Fang VS, Kim MH (1975) Study on maternal, fetal and amniotic human prolactin at term. J Clin Endocrinol Metab 41:1030–1034
278. Shanies DD, Hirschhorn K, New MI (1972) Metabolism of testosterone-^{14}C by cultured human cells. J Clin Invest 51:1459–1468
279. Frandsen VA, Stakeman G (1964) The site of production of oestrogenic hormones in human pregnancy. III. Acta Endocrinol (Copenh) 47:265–276
280. Hausknecht RU, Mandelbaum N (1969) The metabolism of intraamniotically injected dehydroepiandrosterone as a placenta function test. Am J Obstet Gynecol 104:433–435
281. Tabei T, Heinrichs WL (1976) Diagnosis of placental sulfatase deficiency. Am J Obstet Gynecol 124:409–414
282. Dell'Acqua S, Parloti E, Lucisano A, Plotti G, Seri F, Bompiani A (1979) Evaluation of the feto-placental function by means of intraamniotic administration of dehydroepiandrosterone sulfate. J Perinat Med 7:149–159
283. Lehmann WD, Strecker JR (1976) Estrogens in maternal plasma following intra-amniotic injection of (^{3}H)-dehydroepiandrosterone sulfate in mid-pregnancy. J Perinat Med 4:225-260
284. Ylikorkala O, Kauppila A, Rimilä M, Tuimala R (1980) Intraamniotic or intravenous injection of dehydroepiandrosterone sulphate: Simultaneous changes in steroid levels in amniotic fluid and maternal serum. Clin Endocrinol 12:261-267
285. Gurpide E, Schwers J, Welch MT, van de Wiele RL, Lieberman S (1966) Fetal and maternal metabolism of estradiol during pregnancy. J Clin Endocrinol Metab 26:1335–1365
286. Schwers J, Gurpide E, van de Wiele RL, Lieberman S (1967) Urinary metabolite of estradiol and estriol administered intraamniotically. J Clin Endocrinol Metab 27:1403–1408
287. Klopper AJ, Dennis KJ, Farr V (1968) Urinary estriol after intraamniotic injection of estriol sulfate. Br Med J II:158–159
288. Klopper A, Dennis KJ (1969) The urinary excretion of estriol after intraamniotic injection of estriol sulfate as a test of placental function. J Obstet Gynaecol Br Commonw 76:534–537
289. Dennis KG, Farr V, Klopper A (1973) The effect of intraamniotic estriol sulfate on abortion induced by hypertonic saline. J Obstet Gynaecol Br Commonw 80:41–45
290. Klopper A, Farr V, Dennis KJ (1973) The effect of intraamniotic estriol sulfate on uterine contractility at term. J Obstet Gynaecol Br Commonw 80:34–40
291. Lefebvre Y, Marier R, Amyot G, Bolideau R, Hotte R, Raynoult P, Durvehar JG, Lanthier A (1976) Maternal, fetal and intraamniotic hormonal and biological changes resulting from a single dose of hydrocortisone injected in the intraamniotic compartment. Am J Obstet Gynecol 125:609–612
292. Nwosu U, Bolognese R, Stevens V, Wallach E (1976) Maternal steroid levels following intraamniotic cortisol installation in human pregnancy. Gynecol Invest 7:101-102
293. Nwosu UC, Wallach EE, Bolognese RJ (1976) Initiation of labor by intraamniotic cortisol instillation in prolonged human pregnancy. Obstet Gynecol 47:137-142
294. Wu CH, Mennuti MT, Mikhail G (1979) Free and protein-bound steroids in amniotic fluid of mid-pregnancy. Am J Obstet Gynecol 133:666-672

295. Benzie RJ, Doran A, Harkins JL, Jones Owen VM, Porter CJ (1974) Composition of the amniotic fluid and maternal serum in pregnancy. Am J Obstet Gynecol 119:798–810
296. Challis JRG, Benett MJ (1977) Cortisol binding in human amniotic fluid. Am J Obstet Gynecol 129:655–661
297. Caputo MJ, Hosty TA (1974) Further characterization of the sex hormone-binding globulins in amniotic fluid. Am J Obstet Gynecol 118:496–498
298. Siiteri PK, MacDonald PC (1967) The origin of placental estrogen precursors during human pregnancy. Excerpta Med Int Congr Ser 132:726–732
299. Smith R, Klopper A, Hughes G, Wilson G (1979) The compartmental distribution of estrogens and pregnancy specific β_1-glycoprotein. Br J Obstet Gynaecol 86:119–124
300. Shome B, Parlow AF (1976) The primary structure of the hormone-specific, beta subunit of human pituitary luteinizing hormone (hLH). J Clin Endocrinol Metab 42:9–19
301. Clements JA, Reyes FI, Winter JSD, Faiman C (1976) Studies on human sexual development. III. Fetal pituitary and serum, and amniotic fluid concentration of LH, CG, and FSH. J Clin Endocrinol Metab 42:9–19
302. Dattetreyamurty B, Sheth AR, Parundare TV, Companiwalla R, Krishna U (1979) Gonadotropins during second trimester of pregnancy. I. LH and hCG levels in maternal serum and amniotic fluid and their relationship to the sex of the fetus. Acta Endocrinol (Copenh) 91:692–703
303. Ross GT (1974) Gonadotropins and preantral folicular maturation in women. Fertil Steril 25:522–543
304. Schindler AE, Friedrich E (1975) Steroid metabolism of fetal tissues. I. Metabolism of pregnenolone-4-^{14}C by human fetal ovaries. Endokrinologie 65:72–79
305. Reyes FI, Boroditsky RS, Winter JSD, Faiman C (1974) Studies on human sexual development. II. Fetal and maternal serum gonadotropin and sex steroid concentrations. J Clin Endocrinol Metab 38:612–617
306. Berle P (1969) Der Gehalt an chorialem Gonadotropin im Fruchtwasser während der normalen und pathologischen Schwangerschaft. Acta Endocrinol (Copenh) 61:369–377
307. Brunner JA (1951) Distribution of chorionic gonadotropin in the mother and fetus at various stages of pregnancy. J Clin Endocrinol Metab 11:360
308. Crosignani PG, Trojsi L, Attanasio AEM, Lombroso GC (1974) Value of HCG and HCS measurement in clinical practice. Obstet Gynecol 44:673–681
309. Crosignani PG, Nencioni T, Brambati B (1972) Concentration of chorionic gonadotropin and chorionic somatotropin in maternal serum, amniotic fluid and cord blood serum at term. J Obstet Gynaecol Br Commonw 79:122–126
310. Dericks-Tan JSE, Baumann R (1977) Feto-maternale HCG-, HCS- and Prl-Konzentrationen in der perinatalen Periode. Geburtshilfe Frauenheilkd 36:845–851
311. Leudsen van HA: HCG in pathologic pregnancy. Eur .J Obstet Gynecol Reprod Biol 3:137–146
312. Brody S, Carlström G (1965) Human chorionic gonadotropin pattern in serum and its relation to the sex of the fetus. J Clin Endocrinol Metab 25:792–797
313. Kaplan SL, Grumbach MM (1965) Immunoassay for human chorionic "growth hormone-prolactin" in serum and urine. Science 147:751–753
314. Mishell DR, Wide L, Gemzell LA (1963) Immunologic determination of human chorionic gonadotropin in serum. J Clin Endocrinol Metab 23:125–131
315. McGarthy C, Pennington GW (1964) Immunological determination of chorionic gonadotropin in liquor amnii and its application in Rh-incompatibility. Am J Obstet Gynecol 89: 1074–1077
316. Geiger W (1974) Methodik und Ergebnisse radioimmunologischer Bestimmungen von HCG, HCS, STH und TSH aus mütterlichen und kindlichen Körperflüssigkeiten während der Schwangerschaft, Geburt und Wochenbett. Fortschr Geburtshilfe Gynaekol 52:1–120
317. Tallberg T, Ruoslahti E, Ehnholm C (1965) Immunological studies in human placental protein and the purification of human placental lactogen. Ann Med Exp Fenn 43:67–71
318. Josimovich JB (1971) Placental lactogenic hormone. In Fuchs F, Klopper A (eds) Endocrinology of pregnancy. Harper & Row, New York, pp 184–196
319. Tyson JE, Hwang P, Guyda H, Friesen HG (1972) Studies of prolactin secretion in human pregnancy. Am J Obstet Gynecol 113:14–20
320. Hechtermans R, L'Hermite-Balaraux M, Delhaye C, Jacob D, Flamme P (1972) Dosage

radio-immunologique du HPL dans le liquide amniotique prélevé par amniocentèse au voisinage du terme de la gestation. J Gynecol Obstet Biol Reprod (Paris) [Suppl 2] 1: 328-330

321. Berle P (1974) Pattern of the human chorionic somatotropic (HCS) concentration ratio in maternal serum and amniotic fluid during normal pregnancy. Acta Endocrinol (Copenh) 76:364-368
322. Berle P, Schultze-Mosgau H (1974) Das Verhalten des plazentaren Laktogens im mütterlichen Serum und im Fruchtwasser bei Rh-inkompatibilität. Arch Gynaekol 216:284-287
323. Belleville F, Nabet P, Paysant R, Schweitzer A, Landes P (1974) Etude du tous en HCS du plasma et du liquide amniotique au cours du grossesses normals et pathologiques. J Gynecol Obstet Biol Reprod (Paris) 3:883-894
324. Ylikorkala O, Tuimala R (1975) Human placental lactogen (HPL) levels in amniotic fluid. Int J Gynaecol Obstet 13:123-126
325. Weiss RR, Frantz AG, Macri JN, Robins J, Merker JG (1977) Prolactin and human placental lactogen changes in maternal serum and amniotic fluid in midtrimester induced abortions. Am J Obstet Gynecol 129:9-13
326. Lolis D, Konstantinidis K, Papevangelou G, Kaskarelis D (1977) Comparative study of amniotic fluid and maternal blood serum human placental lactogen in normal and prolonged pregnancies. Am J Obstet Gynecol 128:724-726
327. Lolis D, Kaskarelis D (1978) Human placental lactogen levels in normal and toxemic pregnancies. Acta Obstet Gynecol Scand 57:367-369
328. Lolis D, Tzingounis V, Kaskarelis D (1978) Maternal serum and amniotic fluid levels of human placental lactogens in gestational diabetes. Eur J Clin Invest 8:259-260
329. Niven PAR, Ward RHT, Chard T (1974) Human placental lactogen levels in amniotic fluid in rhesus isoimmunization. J Obstet Gynaecol Br Commonw 81:988-990
330. Chez RA, Josimovich JB, Schultz SG (1978) The transfer of human placental lactogen across isolated amnion-chorion. Gynecol Invest 1:312-318
331. Josimovich JB (1978) Hormones in the amniotic fluid. In: Fairweather DVI, Eskes TKAB (eds) Amniotic fluid—Research in clinical application, 2nd edn. Excerpta Medica, Amsterdam, pp 209-223
332. Moser RJ, Hollingsworth DR (1972) Radioimmunoassay of hormone chorionic somatotropin in serum, amniotic fluid and urine. Clin Chem 19:602-607
333. Spellacy WN, Teoh ES, Buhl WC, Birk SA, McCreary SA(1971) Value of human chorionic somatotropin in managing high-risk pregnancies. Am J Obstet Gynecol 109:588-598
334. Wortmann W, Wortmann B, Melchert F, Hepp H (1975) Lecithin/Sphingomyelin-Quotient und HCS im Fruchtwasser. Arch Gynaekol 219:387-388
335. Singer W, Desjardins P, Friesen HG (1970) Human placental lactogen. Obstet Gynecol 36:222-232
336. Ezes H, Wahl P, Deltour G, Robinet G, Chaste F (1973) Le dosage de L'homme chorionique somatomammotrophique au cours de l'isoimmunisation anti-D. J Gynecol Obstet Biol Reprod (Paris) 2:533-537
337. Tescher M, Lemoine JP, Morin P, Merger R (1974) Intérêt du dosage d'HCS plasmatique et amniotique dans l'immunisation rhésus. J Gynecol Obstet Biol Reprod (Paris) 3:1255-1265
338. Altmann P, Kucera H, Sponer J (1975) Zur Abschätzung des kindlichen Risikos durch Bestimmung des Serum-Fruchtwasser-Quotienten von HPL während der Schwangerschaft. Z Geburtshilfe Perinatol 179:278-285
339. Hwang P, Guyda H, Friesen HG (1971) A radioimmunoassay for human prolactin. Proc Natl Acad Sci USA 68:1902
340. Parke L (1973) Detection of prolactin activity by bioassay. J Endocrinol 58:137-138
341. Shani J, Zambelman L, Khazen K, Sulman FG (1970) Mammotrophic and prolactin-like effects of rat and human placental and amniotic fluid. J Endocrinol 46:15-20
341a. Rathnam P, Cederqvist L, Saxena BB (1977) Isolation of prolactin from human amniotic fluid. Biochem Biophys Acta 492:186-196
342. Ben-David M, Rodbard D, Bates RW, Bridson WE, Chrambach A (1973) Human prolactin in plasma, amniotic fluid and pituitary: Identity and characterization by criteria of electrophoresis and isoelectric focusing in polyacrylamide gel. J Clin Endocrinol Metab 36:951-964
343. Ben-David M, Chrambach A (1974) Isolation of isohormones of human prolactin from amniotic fluid. Endocr Res Commun 1:193-210

344. Rogol AD, Chrambach A (1975) Radioiodinated human pituitary and amniotic fluid prolactins with preserved molecular integrity. Endocrinology 97:406–417
345. Ben-David M, Chrambach A (1977) Preparation of bio- and immunoactive human prolactin in milligram amounts from amniotic fluid in 60% yield. Endocrinology 101:250-261
346. Hwang P, Murray JB, Jacobs JW, Niall HD, Friesen HG (1974) Human amniotic prolactin. Purification by affinity chromatography and amino-terminal sequence. Biochemistry 13: 2354–2358
347. Biswass S (1976) Prolactin in amniotic fluid: Its correlation with maternal plasma prolactin. Clin Chem Acta 73:363-367
348. Soria J, Canales ES, Forsbach G, Kardena S, Guzmann V, Zarate A (1977) Relationship of maternal, fetal and amniotic fluid prolacting levels. Ann Endocrinol (Paris) 38:55-59
349. Bigazzi M, Ronga R, Lancranjan I, Ferraro S, Branchoni F, Buzzoni P, Martorana G, Scarcelli GF, Pozo del E (1975) A pregnancy in an acromegalic woman during bromocryptine treatment: Effects on growth hormone and prolactin in the maternal, fetal and amniotic compartments. J Clin Endocrinol Metab 41:1030-1034
350. McMeilly AS, Gilmore D, Jeffery D, Dolbie G, Chard T (1977) The origin of prolactin in amniotic fluid: Fetal or maternal? In: Crosignani PG, Robyn C (eds) Prolactin and human reproduction. Academic Press, London, pp 21-26
351. Golander A, Hurley T, Barett J, Handwerger S (1979) Synthesis of prolactin by human decidua in vitro J Endocrinol 82:263-267
352. Josimovich JB (1977) The role of pituitary prolactin in fetal and amniotic fluid water and salt balance. In: Crosignani PG, Robyn C (eds) Prolactin and hormone reproduction. Academic Press, London, pp 27-36
353. Leontic EA, Tyson JS (1977) Possible osmo-regulatory role for amniotic fluid prolactin. In: Crosignani PG, Robyn C (eds) Prolactin and human reproduction. Academic Press, London, pp 37–45
354. Leontic EA, Schruefer JJ, Andreassen B, Pinto H, Tyson JE (1979) Further evidence for the role of prolactin in human fetal placenta osmo-regulation. Am J Obstet Gynecol 133:435–438
355. Freeman R, Leo-Gur M, Boyar RM, Schulman H (1976) Studies of maternal plasma prolactin and amniotic fluid prolactin. Effects of chlorpromazine and prostaglandin F_2. Obstet Gynecol 47:282-286
356. Mukherjee TK, Tolavarapa TD, Shea B, Bjornson LK, Freedman HL (1978) Amniotic fluid prolactin. NY State J Med 78:2165-2167
357. Hauth JC, Parker CR, MacDonald PC, Porter JC, Johnston JM (1978) A role of fetal prolactin in lung maturation. Obstet Gynecol 51:81–88
358. Josimovich JB, Archer DF (1977) The role of lactogenic hormones in the pregnant women and the fetus. Am J Obstet Gynecol 129:777-780
359. Clements JA, Reyes FI, Winter JSD, Faiman C (1977) Studies on human sexual development. Fetal pituitary serum and amniotic fluid concentrations of prolactin. J Clin Endocrinol Metab 44:408–413
360. Langman MJS, Wormsley KG (1978) Placental diagnosis of primary pituitary dysgenesis. Lancet I:932
361. Ylikorkola D, Kauppila A, Viinikka L (1979) Intraamniotic or intravenous injection of dehydroepiandrosterone sulfate in midgestation: Effect on prolactin level in maternal serum and amniotic fluid. J Clin Endocrinol Metab 49:452–455
362. Ho Yuen B, Cannon W, Wooley S, Charles E (1978) Maternal plasma and amniotic fluid prolactin levels in normal and hypertensive pregnancy. Br J Obstet Gynaecol 85:293-298
363. Schumaker JC, Skoulios G, Eberst B, Elharrar R, Ritter J, Gandar R (1978) Étude de la prolactine au cours de la grossesse; dans le sang maternel et le liquide amniotique. Senologia 3:49–53
364. Schenker JG, Ben-David M, Polishuk WZ (1975) Prolactin in normal pregnancy: Relationship of maternal, fetal and amniotic fluid levels. Am J Obstet Gynecol 123:834–838
365. Chochinov RH, Ketupanya A, Mariz IK, Underwood LE, Daughaday WH (1976) Amniotic fluid reactivity detected by somatomatin C receptor assay: Correlation with growth hormone, prolactin and fetal renal maturation. J Clin Endocrinol Metab 42:983-986
366. Hardt W, Schmidt-Gollwitzer M, Commichan H, Nevinny-Stickel J (1978) Regulation der Prolaktinsekretion in der Schwangerschaft und im Wochenbett. Gynaekol Praxis 2:581-588

367. Tuimala R, Kauppila A, Haapalahti J (1976) ACTH levels in amniotic fluid during pregnancy. Br J Obstet Gynaecol 83:853–856
368. Allen JP, Cook DM, Kendall JW, McGilora R (1973) Maternal-fetal ACTH relationship in man. J Clin Endocrinol Metab 37:230–234
369. Winters AJ, Oliver C, Colston C, MacDonald PC, Porter JC (1974) Plasma ACTH levels in the human fetus and neonate as related to age and parturition. J Clin Endocrinol Metab 39:269–273
370. Miyakawa I, Ikada I, Mayama M (1974) Transport of ACTH across human placenta. J Clin Endocrinol Metab 39:440–442
371. Honda KS, Fuhni Y (1969) Human growth hormone and insulin in the maternal and fetal blood and the amniotic fluid at each month of pregnancy. J Jpn Obstet Gynecol Soc 21: 1133-1134
372. Genetet F, Nabet P, Streiff F, Genetet P, Paysant P, Landes P (1970/71) Determination of human growth hormone (H.G.H.) activity in the amniotic fluid in feto-maternal disease. Ann Ostet Ginecol Med Perinat 92:521-524
373. Gluckman PD, Grumbach MM, Kaplan SL (1980) The human fetal hypothalamus and pituitary gland. In: Tulchinsky D, Ryen KJ (eds) Maternal-fetal endocrinology. Saunders, Philadelphia, pp 196–222
374. Kastrup KW, Anderson HJ, Lebech P (1978) Somatomedin in newborns and the relationship to human chorionic somatotropin and fetal growth. Acta Paediatr Scand 67:757-762
375. Bala RM, Smith GR (1976) Partial chracterization of somatomedin bioactivity in term human amniotic fluid. J Clin Endocrinol Metab 43:907-912
376. Bala RM, Wright C, Bardai A, Smith GR (1978) Somatomedin bioactivity in serum and amniotic fluid during pregnancy. J Clin Endocrinol Metab 46:649–654
377. Zoppetti G, Cottino F, Lombardi M, Bailone C, Cenderelli C, Costa A (1971) A study of maternal and fetal serum and amniotic fluid thyrotropin levels. J Nucl Biol Med 15:116–121
378. Chopra IJ, Crandall BF (1975) Thyroid hormones and thyrotropin in amniotic fluid. N Engl J Med 293:740–743
379. George WF, Rudolph MC (1976) Fetal hypothyroidism and amniotic fluid TSH. N Engl J Med 294:52
380. Roti E, Mahvasi F, Bandini P, Robuschi G, Benassi L, Gnudi A (1979) 3,3,5-triiodothyronine concentrations in amniotic fluid at different stages of pregnancy. J Endocrinol Invest 2: 213–216
381. Osathanondh R, Chopra IJ, Tulchinsky D, Limansky I (1978) Amniotic fluid reverse triiodothyronine in complicated pregnancies. J Clin Endocrinol Metab 46:365–368
382. Etling N, Gehin-Fouque F, Vielh JP, Gautray JP (1979) The iodine content of amniotic fluid and placental transfer of iodinated drugs. Obstet Gynecol 53:376–380
383. Klein AH, Murphy BEP, Artal R, Oddie TH, Fisher DA (1980) Amniotic fluid thyroid hormone concentrations during human gestation. Am J Obstet Gynecol 136:626–630
384. Sack J, Fisher DA, Hobel CJ, Lam R (1975) Thyroxine in human amniotic fluid. J Pediatr 87:364–368
385. Hollingsworth DR, Austin E (1971) Thyroxine derivatives in amniotic fluid. J Pediatr 79:923–929
386. Morley JE, Bashore RA, Reed A, Carlson HE, Hershman JM (1979) Thyrotropin-releasing hormone and thyroid hormones in amniotic fluid. Am J Obstet Gynecol 134:581–584
387. Klein AH, Hobel CJ, Sack J, Fisher DA (1978) Effect of intraamniotic fluid thyroxine injection on fetal serum and amniotic fluid iodothyronine concentration. J Clin Endocrinol Metab 47:1034–1037
388. Meinhold H, Wenzel KW, Dudenhausen JW, Saling E (1976) Reverse triiodothyronine and thyroxine in amniotic fluid. Acta Endocrinol [Suppl 204] 82:28
389. Burman KD, Read J, Dimond RC, Strum D, Wright FD, Patow W, Earel JM, Wartofsky L (1976) Measurements of 3,3,5-triiodothyronine (rT_3),3,3-L-diiodothyronine, T_3 and T_4 in amniotic fluid and in cord and maternal serum. J Clin Endocrinol Metab 43:1351-1354
390. Herle van AJ, Young RT, Fisher DA, Uller RP, Brinkman CR (1975) Intra-uterine treatment of a hypothyroid fetus. J Clin Endocrinol Metab 40:474–477
391. Redding RA, Douglas WH, Stein M (1971) Thyroid hormone influence upon lung surfactant metabolism. Science 175:994–996
392. Mashiach S, Barkai G, Sack J, Stern E, Goldman B, Busch M, Serr DM (1978) Enhance-

ment of fetal lung maturity by intraamniotic administration of thyroid hormone. Am J Obstet Gynecol 130:289-293
393. Filetti S, Camus M, Rodeschi F, Delange F, Vigueri R, Ermans AM (1977) Decreased reverse triiodothyronine (rT_3) concentration in amniotic fluid in fetal hypothyroidism. Arch Dis Child 52:430–431
394. Lightner ES, Fismer DA, Giles H, Woolfenden J (1977) Intraamniotic injection of thyroxine (T_4) to a human fetus. Am J Obstet Gynecol 127:487–490
395. Weimer S, Scharf JI, Bolognese RJ, Librizzi RJ (1980) Antinatal diagnosis and treatment of fetal goiter. J Reprod Med 24:39-42
396. Landau H, Sack J, Frucht H, Plati Z, Hochner-Celnikier D, Rosenmann A (1980) Amniotic fluid 3,3',5'triiodothyronine in the detection of congenital hypothyroidism. J Clin Endocrinol Metab 50:799–801
397. Wu S-Y, Chopra IJ, Nakamura Y, Salomon DH, Benett LR (1976) A radioimmunoassay for measurement of 3,3'-diiodothyronine (T_2). J Clin Endocrinol Metab 43:682–685
398. Dawood MY, Ylikorkala O, Trivedi D, Fuchs F (1979) Oxytocin in maternal circulation and amniotic fluid during pregnancy. J Clin Endocrinol Metab 49:429–434
399. Dawood MY, Raghavan KS, Pociask C, Fuchs F (1978) Oxytocin in human pregnancy and parturition. Obstet Gynecol 51:138-143
400. Seppälä M, Aho I, Tissari A, Ruoslahti E (1979) Radioimmunoassay of oxytocin in amniotic fluid, fetal urine and meconium during late pregnancy and delivery. Am J Obstet Gynecol 114:788-795
401. Gerlini G, Fallucca F, Pachi A, Bresadola M, Ossicini C, Russo A, Sbraccia (1977) Amniotic fluid insulin and glucagon in normal pregnancy and pregnancy complicated by rhesus isoimmunization. Br J Obstet Gynaecol 84:819–823
402. Pearlman M, Gordin M (1978) Glucagon, insulin and glucose in amniotic fluid. Br J Obstet Gynaecol 85:479
403. Sperling MA, Christensen RA, Artal A, Mies P (1977) The nature and significance of amniotic fluid glucagon. Pediatr Res 11:412
404. Weiss PAM (1979) Die Überwachung des Ungeborenen bei Diabetes mellitus an Hand von Fruchtwasserinsulinwerten. Wien Klin Wochenschr 91:293-304
405. Spellacy WN, Buhl WC, Bradley B, Holzinger KK (1973) Maternal, fetal and amniotic fluid levels of glucose, insulin and growth hormone. Obstet Gynecol 41:323-331
406. Draisey TF, Gagneja GL, Thibert RJ (1977) Pulmonary surfactant and amniotic fluid insulin. Obstet Gynecol 50:197-199
407. Tzingounis V, Katsilambros N, Prevedourakis C, Papaevangelou G (1977) Insulin levels in the amniotic fluid and in maternal and fetal blood. J Reprod Med 19:259-261
408. Hall RT, Rhodes PG, Newman RL (1977) Glucose disappearance in infants of diabetic mothers. Relationship to lowest neonatal blood glucose and mniotic fluid insulin. Early Hum Dev 1:257-264
409. Tzingounis V, Lolis D, Kaskarelis D (1978) Amniotic fluid, maternal and fetal blood insulin in overweight pregnant women. Horm Res 9:249-253
410. Weiss PAM, Lichtenegger W, Winter R, Pürstner P (1978) Insulin levels in amniotic fluid. management of pregnancy in diabetes. Obstet Gynecol 51:393-398
411. Casper DJ, Benjamin F (1970) Immunoreactive insulin in amniotic fluid. Obstet Gynecol 35:389-393
412. Newman RL, Tutera G (1976) The glucose-insulin ratio in amniotic fluid. Obstet Gynecol 47:599-601
413. Weiss PAM (1978) Der Fruchtwasserinsulingehalt als fetaler Parameter zur Stoffwechselführung der schwangeren Diabetikerin. In: Irsigler K, Regal H, Brändle J (eds) Diabetes-Probleme in der Schwangerschaft. Urban & Schwarzenberg, München, pp 117-120
414. Newman RL (1977) The relationship of amniotic fluid insulin levels and the lecithin-sphingomyelin ratio. Int J Gynaecol Obstet 15:17-19
415. Vidnes J, Finne H (1977) Immunoreactive insulin in amniotic fluid from Rh-immunized women. Biol Neonate 31:1-6
416. Greco AV, Rebuzzi AG, Bellat U, Serri F, Altomonta L, Manna R, Ghirlanda (1980) Fetal origin of amniotic fluid insulin in the human fetus. Clin Endocrinol 12:67-70
417. Mitnick MA, Chieffo V, Gibbons JM, Hurley KJ (1974) Isolation of TRH and LRH from human amniotic fluid and their in vitro binding to human chorio-amniotic membranes (abstr) In: Program 56th Ann. Meeting of the Endocrine Society, Atlanta

418. Bassini RM, Utinger RD (1972) The preparation and specificity of antibody to thyrotropin releasing hormone. Endocrinology 90:722-727
419. Robinson AG, Archer DF, Tolstoi LF (1973) Neurophysin in women during oxytocin-related events. J Clin Endocrinol Metab 37:645-649
420. Gauthray JP, Jolivet A, Vielh JP, Guillemin R (1977) Presence of immunoassayable β-endorphin in human amniotic fluid: Elevation in cases of fetal distress. Am J Obstet Gynecol 129:211-212
421. Wilkes MM, Stewart RD, Bruni JF, Quigley ME, Yen SSC, Ling N, Chrétien M (1980) A specific homologous radioimmunoassay for human β-endorphin: Direct measurement in biological fluids. J Clin Endocrinol Metab 50:309-315
422. Ances IG, Pomerantz SH (1974) Serum concentrations of β-melanocyte-stimulating hormone in human pregnancy. Am J Obstet Gynecol 119:1062-1068
423. Pschera H, Björkhem I, Carlström K, Lantto O, Lunell NO, Persson B, Somell C, Stangenberg M, Wagner J (1979) Total cortisol and L/S ratio in amniotic fluid in late pregnancy complicated by diabetes mellitus. Horm Metab Res 11:612-615
424. Fencl M, Koos B, Tulchinsky D (1980) Origin of corticosteroids in amniotic fluid. J Clin Endocrinol Metab 50:431-436
425. Laatikainen TJ, Peltonen JI (1980) Amniotic fluid estriol, estriol precursors and pregnanediol in intrauterine growth retardation. J Steroid Biochem 13:265-269
426. Sulcova J, Jirasek JE, Dvorák P, Starka L (1980) The development of the androgen metabolising activity in the human amniotic epithelium. J Steroid Biochem 12:84-93
427. Hustin J, Van Cauwenberghe JR, Reuter A, Franchimont P, Lambotte R (1980) Prolactine placentaire: Immunocytochimie. Ann Endocrinol (Paris) 41:141-142
428. Burman KD, Wright FD, Smallridge RC, Green B, Georges LP, Wartofsky L (1978) Radioimmunoassay for 3′,5′-diiodothyronine. J Clin Endocrinol Metab 47:1059-1064
429. Chopra IJ, Geola F, Solomon DH, Maciel RMB (1978) 3′,5′-Diiodothyronine in health and disease: Studies by a radioimmunoassay. J Clin Endocrinol Metab 47:1198-1207
430. Maciel RMB, Chopra IJ, Ozawa Y, Geola F, Solomon DH (1979) A radioimmunoassay for measurement of 3′,5′-diiodothyronine. J Clin Endocrinol Metab 49:399-405
431. Chopra IJ (1980) A radioimmunoassay for measurement of 3′-monoiodothyronine. J Clin Endocrinol Metab 51:117-123
433. Kraan GPB, Derks HJGM, Drayer NM (1980) Quantification of polar glucocorticosteroids in the urine of pregnant and nonpregnant women: a comparison with 6α-hydroxylated metabolites of cortisol in newborn urine and amniotic fluid. J Clin Endocrinol Metab 51:754-758
434. Rosenberg SM, Maslar IA, Riddick DH (1980) Decidual production of prolactin in late gestation. Further evidence for a decidual source of amniotic fluid prolactin. Am J Obstet Gynecol 138:681-685
435. Granet M, Sharf M, Weissman BA (1980) Humoral endorphin in human body fluids during pregnancy. Gynecol Obstet Invest 11:214-218

Subject Index

Other Volumes in This Series:

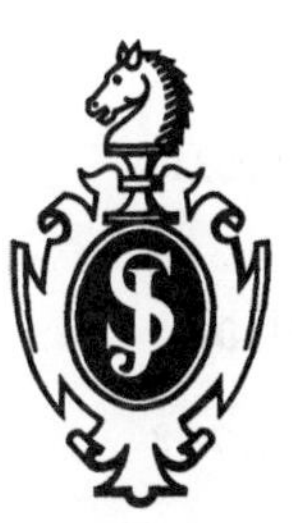

Springer-Verlag
Berlin
Heidelberg
New York

Volume 23: E. Flückiger, E. Del Pozo, K. v. Werder
Prolactin
Physiology, Pharmacology and Clinical Findings
1982. 54 figures, 14 tables. X, 224 pages. ISBN 3-540-11071-2

Volume 22: D. T. Krieger
Cushing's Syndrome
1982. 27 figures in 42 separate illustrations (some in color)
IX, 142 pages. ISBN 3-540-10811-4

Volume 21: A. E. Schindler
Hormones in Human Amniotic Fluid
1982. 23 figures, 133 tables. XII, 158 pages. ISBN 3-540-10810-6

Volume 20: R. Volpé
Auto-immunity in the Endocrine System
1981. 32 figures, 15 tables. X, 187 pages. ISBN 3-540-10677-4

Volume 19: P. Mauvais-Jarvis, F. Kuttenn, I. Mowszowicz
Hirsutism
1981. 32 figures, 10 tables. XI, 110 pages. ISBN 3-540-10509-3

Volume 18: I. J. Chopra
Triiodothyronines in Health and Disease
With a Contribution by V. Cody
1981. 76 figures, 18 tables. IX, 145 pages. ISBN 3-540-10400-3

Volume 17: J. Chayen
The Cytochemical Bioassay of Polypeptide Hormones
1980. 72 figures, 7 tables. XIV, 208 pages. ISBN 3-540-10040-7

Volume 16: J. E. A. McIntosh, R. P. McIntosh
Mathematical Modelling and Computers in Endocrinology
1980. 73 figures, 57 tables. XII, 337 pages. ISBN 3-540-09693-0

Volume 15: A. T. Cowie, I. A. Forsyth, I. C. Hart
Hormonal Control of Lactation
1980. 64 figures, 7 tables. XIV, 275 pages. ISBN 3-540-09680-9

Volume 14: J. H. Clark, E. J. Peck, Jr.
Female Sex Steroids
Receptors and Function
1979. 116 figures, 18 tables. XII, 245 pages. ISBN 3-540-09375-3

Volume 13: H. F. De Luca
Vitamin D – Metabolism and Function
1979. 14 figures. VIII, 80 pages. ISBN 3-540-09182-3

Volume 12:
Glucocorticoid Hormone Action
Editors: J.D.Baxter, G.G.Rousseau
1979. 176 figures, 58 tables. XIX, 638 pages. ISBN 3-540-08973-X

Volume 11: S.Ohno
Major Sex-Determining Genes
1979. 34 figures, 6 tables. XIII, 140 pages. ISBN 3-540-08965-9

Volume 10: W.I.P.Mainwaring
The Mechanism of Action of Androgens
1977. 12 figures, 17 tables. XI, 178 pages. ISBN 3-540-07941-6

Volume 9: R.E.Mancini
Immunologic Aspects of Testicular Function
1976. 36 figures, 8 tables. IX, 114 pages. ISBN 3-540-07496-1

Volume 8: E.Gurpide
Tracer Methods in Hormone Research
1975. 35 figures. XI, 188 pages. ISBN 3-540-07039-7

Volume 7: E.W.Horton
Prostaglandins
1972. 97 figures. XI, 197 pages. ISBN 3-540-05571-1

Volume 6: K.Federlin
Immunopathology of Insulin
Clinical and Experimental Studies
1971. 53 figures. XIII, 185 pages. ISBN 3-540-05408-1

Volume 5: J.Müller
Regulation of Aldosterone Biosynthesis
1971. 19 figures. VII, 137 pages. ISBN 3-540-05213-5

Volume 4: U.Westphal
Steroid-Protein Interactions
1971. 144 figures. XIII, 567 pages. ISBN 3-540-05313-3

Volume 3: F.G.Sulman
Hypothalamic Control of Lactation
In collaboration with numerous experts.
1970. 58 figures. XII, 235 pages. ISBN 3-540-04973-8

Volume 2: K.B.Eik-Nes, E.C.Horning
Gas Phase Chromatography of Steroids
1968. 85 figures. XV, 382 pages. ISBN 3-540-04277-6

Volume 1: S.Ohno
Sex Chromosomes and Sex-linked Genes
1967. 33 figures. X, 192 pages. ISBN 3-540-03934-1

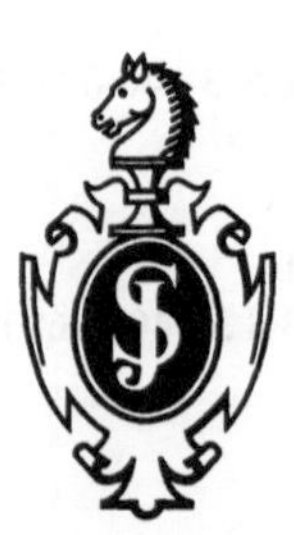

Springer-Verlag
Berlin
Heidelberg
New York